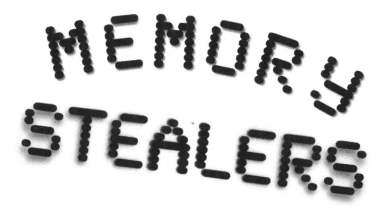

MEMORY STEALERS

By Connie Rogers

Certified Integrative Health & Brain Health Coach

Disclaimer: The content of this book is for general instruction only. Each person's physical emotional and spiritual condition is unique. The instruction in this book is not intended to replace or interrupt the readers relationship with a physician or other professional. Please consult your doctor for matters pertaining to your specific health and dietary needs.

Connie Rogers, Published Author of *Path to a Healthy Mind & Body* and *Fat Vegan*

Now brings you…

Memory Stealers!

Memory Stealers

Table of Contents

Memory Stealers

Special Acknowledgments

Special thanks to the following for their dedication, expertise, and support that helped make the creation of this book possible.

A Big Hug & Thank You to the following:

Claude Fennema PhD / Artist and Owner of Madsen's Photo Service LLC. Thank you for your expertise in lighting up my book cover and capturing a fantastic photo of me for my back cover!

Dr. Daniel Amen is the chief executive officer and medical director of Amen Clinics. Dr Amen is double board certified by the American Board of Psychiatry and Neurology in General Psychiatry and Child and Adolescent Psychiatry, and brain injury specialist, who shaped my life, informed my work, and made this book possible.

Allen Rogers/ Design of book template. Tons of organizing went into this template! I couldn't have finished without your help.

About The Author

My passion is helping my readers take simple, daily 'bite size steps' toward wellness. My love is to educate, and empower people to create long-lasting, sustainable changes, so they can see and taste how good wellness feels. In my world, as a Holistic Chef, food is art. It's a dance through the world rich in colors and textures, unlocking the wellness within. Food is a current affair with sweet and pungent taste and seemingly infinite possibilities. There's a silent joy in preparing a meal that tantalizes taste buds and listening to the ooh's and ah's from others dining with me.

As an Integrative Health Coach, I share with you thousands of hours of reading journals so you can be informed. Also included are stories of friends and entertainers that have touched my life. I feel honored to give them a space on my tablet because they have a place in my heart.

Why I decided to write *Memory Stealers* is my concern for how most view brain health. After a certain age, both men and women have come to accept *losing their mind* as a normal part of aging. However, it doesn't have to be that way. If we were to address some of the many symptoms involved, instead of just managing them, we'd give rise and permission to understand *Memory Stealers*.

And, it's in this awareness we can make an impact on our life or someone we love.

My relationship with Alzheimer's first began many years ago with my father's diagnosis. As a teenager I already suspected there was something amiss before I ventured out on my own.

My father was about 50 years old when he started losing his mind. His moods were always erratic. His comfort foods included coffee, tons of pastrami sandwiches, donuts, coke syrup, and a bowl of ice cream before bed. However truth be told, he was *NEVER* comforted. He was full of anxiety, and suffered from insomnia and constipation most of the time. He unknowingly traumatized himself and all who had the pleasure to know him. In the end, it was his lifestyle that seriously eroded his mind, and cancer eroded his body.

This is not a fix all book but a wake up call to open conversations about how illnesses don't just show up one day. It takes years with ongoing habits and events to progress.

Memory Stealers is extensively researched and referenced.

Each URL I provided has other scientific studies used to validate and verify the quotes, statistics, points and findings. This is how you can have access to hundreds of studies referencing and supporting the positions in my book. These are all active as of February 2020.

Connie Rogers <u>faces@vail.net</u>

"As teenagers, we may have an excellent attention span in class but become indifferent about handing in our homework. At the end of the semester we leave it to the teacher to decide whether we receive a passing grade.

I find it similar when we eat tons of crap! We may become lazy, even lethargic, never participating in self-care or the everyday ritual of consuming nutrient rich foods. Then we visit our doctor for a checkup. We sit and nervously await for the results of that exam, crossing our fingers before a failing grade appears." Connie Rogers

Memory Stealers

Foreword

I have known Connie for 4 years now through her engaging ability to write about real issues that affect our everyday lives. Her new book, *Memory Stealers*, delves deep into the darkness, and delusional mysteries that millions are facing today.

It's a brilliant way of addressing: why memories leave us. The authors in-depth research is backed by over 30 years of application, since her father passed. Connie makes awareness easy, with power notes and digestible tips, throughout her book!

One haunting point that hits home with me is how many of us buy into the *illusions* of products that are somehow going to fix us, when they are designed to keep us sick? Believe me, you'll have NO regrets reading this book presented here by a very passionate author. Once we become aware of events that *steal memories*, we can make conscience choices to avoid losing everything that makes us who we are.

This book provides 'You' the reader with an alternative look into some commonly misunderstood conditions.
FEEL EMPOWERED instead of hopeless!

Thank you Connie, for sharing your inspiring knowledge with others.

Antonio K Starow
Professional Chef & Founder E Bubble Life Magazine

Citations/Index/Resources- footnotes included in back of book!

ISBN: 978-0-578-65119-4

Printed in the United States of America

Connie Rogers is an author/writer of over 300 blogs in dozens of respected online magazines and health sites around the world.

Her books include:
Path to a Healthy Mind & Body
Fat Vegan
Memory Stealers

Chapter Contributor in: *The Book of Success*

http://voilasuccess.com/index.php/products-page/inspirational/the-book-of-success-2/

Chapter Contributor in: *Creating The Life You Want*

http://voilasuccess.com/index.php/products-page/well-being/creating-your-life-dieting-and-physical-fitness/

To contact the author, visit websites:

 BiteSizePieces.net

SkinHealthFromWithin.com

This Book is dedicated to my best friend Sherry

"It is much more important to know what sort of a patient has a disease than what sort of disease a patient has." William Osler

Introduction

It seems everywhere I look there's mental illness. I feel that some type of alien mentality has invaded this planet. People have lost their minds. From cars chasing each other off the road to employees going postal when they are terminated from jobs. From jet pilots addicted to depression, drama, and chaos, to angry, abusive and stressed out couples. From chemicals in our water, food and air, to injecting pain killers in our arm. From teenagers suffering brain injuries in football games, to school administrators suffering with alcohol addictions. From women frequenting toxic nail salons, to the billion dollar carcinogenic makeup industry.

Truth be told we are dying younger, dying to look good, dying to feel good, dying to smell good, dying to increase libido, and dying to sleep better. However, in reality our mental health is suffering. It seems the more we suffer the easier and more interesting our story becomes when we share it with friends and fans.

Statistics show women outnumber men two to one with *Memory Stealers*, frustration, depression, exhaustion and confusion. In order to change statistics we must change the way we find comfort.

Empowerment clears the path of confusion. What we gain with change is power, strength, flexibility and peace of mind when we get to the heart of *uncomfortable.*

Memory Stealers is designed to get us thinking, how did we come this far? Why are we poisoning our children? Why are we poisoning our world? How do we recover*?*

Memory Stealers has the answers!

If you know *Memory Stealers* you may be able to come to your own defense.

Memory Stealers touches everyone's life differently.

*First, you have to know who you are
and where are you going!*

Chapter 1

The Making Of Mental Illness

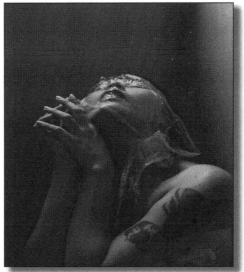

Alzheimer's, Allow Me to Introduce Myself!

"The earth has the ability to clear out the old and bring in the new with hurricanes, floods and fires. After devastations, new growth appears. It seems to the inquisitive mind somehow destruction causes growth. As with humans, our bodies have an innate ability to heal from a break down, renew and regrow cells, regulate stress, and eliminate the trash. But, first, we must get shaken to our core." CR

Alzheimer's is a billion dollar business. Almost seventy-five million cases are estimated to occur in 2030 and 131.5 million in 2050. (1)

Alterations in the gut microbiome may play a pathophysiological role in human brain diseases, including autism spectrum disorder, anxiety, depression, and Alzheimer's. (2)

Every few seconds someone gets diagnosed with Alzheimer's or Dementia. According to the journal of Alzheimer's Disease, Alzheimer's is a metabolic disease in which brain glucose and energy production are impaired. (3)

In addition, they say, "white matter degeneration and demyelination plays a role in Alzheimer's."(4) This leads us to blame toxins and poor nutrition as causes of myelin destruction.

Some studies list contributors to Alzheimer's, such as sex steroid hormones and obesity, but never list strategies for preventing it. (5)

In 2017 a report from the Alzheimer's Association International Conference claims stress and poverty can increase African Americans risk for Alzheimer's Disease.(5a)

"Dramatic studies reveal diffuse amyloid plaques and inflammation in the brains of children and young adults are attributed to residing in places with the worse air quality."[6]

And since it's not common knowledge to what's killing our memories, Alzheimer's can be present 30-40 years before an actual diagnosis is made!

But, somehow, science left out that Alzheimer's is a physical, mental, and all encompassing emotional disorder, metamorphosing *you* into someone you've never seen or heard before in your life!

Memory Stealers devastates your caregiver, as you disappear he holds on tight before he fades away. In the U.S., we now know many strategies to prevent *Memory Stealers*. Whether we pay attention is a different story.

Memory Stealers

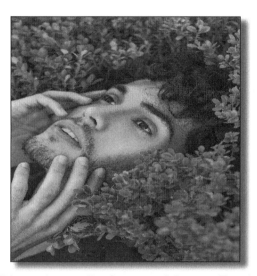

The Physiologically Stressed Brain Epidemic

We panic most days, showing up as if anxiety is all that's left of our brain! We can't think straight, let alone keep our moods in check. Before work we visit our favorite coffee shop to stop that headache and after work, we frequent our favorite sushi bar to de-stress. We slurp, drink and converse, pop antibiotics for sinus infections and use sleeping pills before the night ends. We're high on stimulants and low on energy. The term 'burn out' can be described as 'system sludge'. Blood flow slows and so does brain activity. We're scrambling to get our MoJo back.

Children are growing up on Adderall with additional doses of other stimulants. Amphetamine's, such as Adderall, are neurotoxic. Side-effects include poor moods and changes in circadian rhythms, plus weaknesses in the cardiac system and gastrointestinal system. After they reach adulthood, they've developed improved tolerance for stronger drugs and are locked into mental patterns which can be hard to break later on in life.

I believe a stressed brain, and deep-seated anger begins on our forks and in our homes creating mental instability. It's not only found in our nervous system, it's in our digestive system, integumentary system, and endocrine system. It takes up residence in our hearts, microbiome, bones and frequently entangles our memories. It's what keeps us from sleeping, learning, relating, loving or contemplating a way out.

Anger feeds abuse and mental instability. One example is, when a child becomes a bully. When we take a look at the anger and abuse they endure we would understand why they are abusive. Today we see instances where bullies actually kill classmates on school buses.

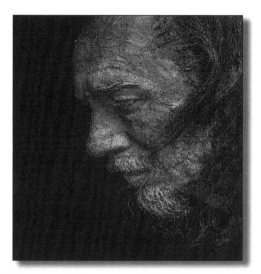

The Many Faces Of Mental Illness

Our brain controls every thought and action we have, including memories, speech, movement and more. CR

My neighbor, Susan, suffered with panic attacks, muscle spasms, and depression. She also ate poorly. Her prescribed medications left her, most days, with memory problems, paranoia, fatigue, confusion and increased depression. She passed away a few years ago in my arms.

Susan took Clonazepam for panic and anxiety disorders. "Benzodiazepine use is associated with an increased risk for Alzheimer's disease,"(77) especially at the end of a five-year period following the initial prescription. (88)

Tizanidine was used for muscle spasticity. This made her depression worse and caused liver damage, respiratory problems, dizziness, and hallucinations. She screamed in pain most days.

Carbamazepine was used for nerve pain and neuropathy. Besides confusion, side-effects included muscle aches and more liver troubles.

Gabapentin was taken for neuropathic pain. Besides memory loss, aggression and coordination issues, she experienced major liver injury, IBS, and kidney problems.

Anytime she felt the flu coming on, she took Tamiflu® which caused more neuropsychiatric side-effects including delusions and delirium. (78)

➡"Four out of every *ten* patients are harmed during primary and ambulatory health care. The most detrimental errors are related to diagnosis, prescriptions and the use of medicines."(79)

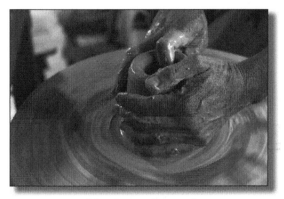

My Best Friend

It's life's illusions I recall. I really don't know life at all!
Joni Mitchell

A note from my best friend.

"Our lives are different now than they were when we first became friends. That's why it's important that we make an effort to stay close. Even though things have changed, I still want you to be an important part of my life and I hope you'll want me to be a part of yours. Let's try to stay close because I don't ever want to drift away from you. Through all the good and the bad, if you ever need me, I'll be there. Love you!"

9

Friends can change each others brain chemistry. My best friend and I believed we were sisters from a past lifetime. We instantly became friends at work. Every time Elvis Presley performed in Las Vegas we were there. We were pregnant together, had our babies born a month apart from each other, took our families camping together, where I learned how to waterski. We celebrated many holidays and birthdays together, cooked together, and ate burritos, tacos, and drank homemade margaritas together. We danced together, created dozens of art projects together, had our children in the same high school together, attended weddings and funerals together. She even became a customer when I opened my first day spa.

We each had our own reasons to break down. I suffered with ulcerative colitis going through a gnarly divorce and a stress filled home life. She lost her son in a swimming pool accident. She also suffered with asthma and sciatica pain most of her life.

She was treated by the best doctors and received the top of the line medications to keep her within a manageable level of pain. Through all the ups and downs, we partied anyway! We lived and loved, followed our dreams, and shared our passions.

This year, I found out my best friend has Alzheimer's and is in hospice.

Friends believe in each other forever! Now, as she loses her mind, a piece of me disappears. **Forever**!

Memory Stealers

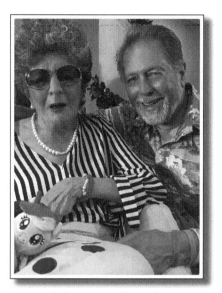

A Loving Couple

About 5 years ago, my friend went on a vacation with his wife and while they were there, his wife became ill with pneumonia. He swiftly rushed her to the hospital. The medical professionals worked feverishly providing treatments and therapies to help her recover.

He feels he left a part of his wife there in the hospital. He describes it as 'she did an about face' and didn't come home the same person he once knew. She went into the hospital walking and talking fine, but had breathing problems. She came out of the hospital in a wheel chair! It seems Chlamydia pneumonia went unnoticed. In his words, "they got back home and went to their doctor who diagnosed his wife with Alzheimer's and gave her medications to take. For months she didn't get any better and so he researched, only to find that the side-effects of the medicines given were causing more confusion and forgetfulness."

In the beginning she spoke a little bit and still walked a bit, but over about a year she lost all of her abilities to walk and talk. Since then, Jose has been with her 24 hours a day. He only sleeps about 3 or 4 hours a night. He's her primary caregiver.

Below is my interview with my friend Jose.

"It's very important to have a routine. Everyday we do pretty much the same routine she's used to doing. She never complains. We start the day with physical therapy to keep her muscles toned. Twice a day we do 2 to 3 hours of physical therapy on fingers, arms, and legs to keep them active. Then, we've added PEMF therapy which has helped tremendously. PEMF therapy accelerates wound healing and improves microcirculation. (79a) She had developed gangrene in her toes and the doctor wanted to amputate both of her legs above the knees. Two weeks after PEMF therapy the gangrene started to disappear and there was no longer any need for amputation. Two months later, she turned and looked me straight in the eye and said: "Hello."

"My way of thinking is to do the best I can every day and I'm happy with that. I take care of her with lots of love and dedication. I do her hair, her makeup, dress her nicely, and put on her favorite pearls. I'm happy to have her for as long as I can." Jose

Memory Stealers

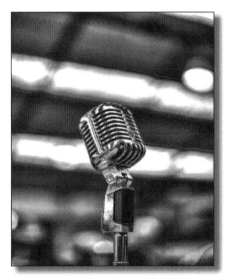

Entertaining Depression

My story begins as a teenager completely mesmerized by certain celebrities, musicians, and entertainers. I thought myself very fortunate to grow up in the age of real music and talented comedians. It couldn't get any better! My favorites included and still are The Beatles, The Eagles, Linda Ronstadt, Jay Leno, Carol Burnett, Robin Williams, and Vivien Leigh, just to name a few.

Love songs and comedy, it seems, are more lovable with a twist of sadness! It happens so often in the entertainment business. My love for Williams and Ronstadt grew because they were within my age range, and I was in awe of their brilliance. They both came to LA to pursue their careers. While I attended the school of hard knocks in L.A., Williams attended Juilliard.

Ronstadt grew up surrounded by music. She had an impeccable voice; not one could emulate. Both of these beautiful people suffered from depression, and they both experimented with cocaine. In an interview, Ronstadt talked about *love* and said, "people commit suicide without it because they can't make an intimate connection with someone. You need that, or else it's religion or drugs. And drugs, there's no way out of that!"

Ronstadt had her nose cauterized twice. After that, she didn't use cocaine anymore.

Williams said his wake up call from cocaine abuse was when John Belushi died at age 33 of a drug overdose.

Today Ronstadt suffers from Parkinson's. Williams suffered from Lewy body dementia, insomnia, anxiety, and an impaired sense of smell. "He was severely depressed before he took his own life." (78a) Incidentally, both Alzheimer's and Lewy body show signs of temporal lobe atrophy. (78b)

Parkinson is described as a neuropsychiatric illness and associated with Neurodegeneration. Lewy bodies is described as a neurodegenerative disorder, having damaged neurotransmitters and progressive cognitive decline. (78c)

Memory Stealers

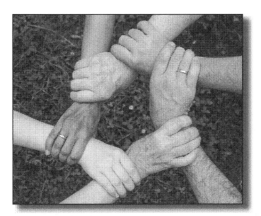

Under Our Skin & Into Our Brain

> The skin is an endocrine organ. (18) Cells in our skin, brain, and gut are linked by a common embryonic origin.

Our skin is intricately connected to our nervous system. In fact the skin, the nervous system and the immune system are not independent systems but are closely associated and use the same language of neurotransmitters. (19) "Our skin is a highly biologically active organ capable of chemical metabolism."(19b) This is where toxins can make their way into our organs not only through our gut or sinuses, but through our skin.

Psychogenic Itching & Memory Stealers

Psychogenic itching and picking of the skin is mostly found in women and associated with psychiatric disorders. These M*emory Stealers'* disorders include depression, stress, anxiety, mania, psychosis, social instability, and more. Studies suggest Tricyclic antidepressants (maprotiline) be used to calm the itch. Unfortunately, side-effects from maprotiline are not pleasant. They increase depression, anxiety, panic attacks, sleep problems, memory problems, or confusion. [19a] Crazy making as it may sound, tricyclics are also prescribed to reduce pain transmission through the spinal cord. [29a]

Microorganisms & Alzheimer's

Fungi As recently as 2018, a study showed the involvement of fungi in Alzheimer's following a long-held suspicion that they may play a role. [29]

Today, there is compelling evidence for the existence of fungal proteins in brain samples from Alzheimer's disease patients. [30] Another study showed Aβ peptide, a cardinal feature of Alzheimer's pathology, could specifically induce Aβ mediated inflammatory activity with Candida albicans. [31]

Bacteria Science has made great strides and hypothesized that amyloids produced by gut bacteria can pass through the gut tract and accumulate in the brain. (32) This means, "Chronic bacterial infections could lead to amyloid deposition and contribute to Aβ deposition in Alzheimer's."(33) One example of this is when the bacteria spirochetes initiate a cascade of events leading to an inflammatory condition of the central nervous system. (34) Another study concluded, spirochetes can slowly progress to dementia and brain atrophy. (35)

Chlamydia Chlamydia pneumoniae is an intracellular bacterium, an airborne organism that normally enters into the body through the mucosa of the respiratory tract and is reported in central nervous system disorders such as Alzheimer's. (36) This organism can silently infect other cells in the body and is found as a risk factor in heart disease and stroke. (36a)

Lupus Systemic lupus erythematosus may lead to the progressive compromise of neural activity. (37) "Findings indicate that a marker of neuronal degeneration, are clearly increased in lupus patients showing signs of dementia." (38-39-40)

Lyme "Residents of Europe have been exposed to Lyme Disease spirochetes as far back as 1884, concurrent with the oldest record of apparent human infection."[41] Lyme Disease or Borrelia can be found causal in neurological disorders but can also cause psychiatric symptoms such as anxiety, panic attacks, poor memory, and suicidal thoughts. [42] Other psychiatric reactions that have been associated with Lyme Disease include dementia, schizophrenia, OCD, paranoia, fatigue and major depressive disorders. [43-44] In 1986 a study found Borrelia in the brains of patients dying with dementia. [45]

➡ I've seen individuals use antibiotics for 3 to 7 months to tackle Lyme. But antibiotics of this length may only serve to drive "Lyme Critters" deeper into the tissue, organs, brain, and bones. Using holistic/alternative methods and protocols are influential to their demise.

Viruses & Alzheimer's

Beta-amyloid autoantibodies (a protein produced by the immune system) are common and are related to herpes simplex virus and numerous other viruses, eventually infecting neurons in Alzheimer's Disease. (21-22) If we choose to use prescribed medications for herpes, we can also be risking increased cognitive decline from the side-effects they cause.

This gives rise to the theory, when we damage our skin, we also damage our brain. (23) Give it a little bit of thought, and you'll see it's true. For example, herpes virus enters thru the skin, lingers in the nervous system of the skin, and can cause central nervous system illnesses eventually damaging brain cells, thus playing a causative role in Alzheimer's. (24)

Hepatitis C virus (HCV), an infection located in the liver, is not just about dirty needles or shellfish. HCV infection is associated with gut dysbiosis (poor gut microbiome). Globally its estimated 71 million are suffering. (48) This virus may increase our risk for dementia as it damages our liver. (26)

Epstein-Barr Virus (EBV), known as mononucleosis, is also linked to cognitive decline.(27)

Additionally, Human Papilloma Virus, from skin to skin contact, shows signs for oxidative stress and inflammation linked with Alzheimer's. Unfortunately, scientist just continues to search for new drugs. (28)

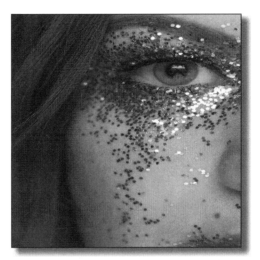

Brain Drain & Memory Loss

Our brain is an energetically demanding organ, less we forget to pay attention.CR

"Memory loss is the key feature of a majority of neurodegenerative diseases." Neurodegeneration is associated with inflammation and referred to as neuronal cell loss. (175) Notably, "there is also an association between noradrenergic depletion and neurodegeneration, which includes Alzheimer's."(176)

"Noradrenergic dysfunction contributes to brain drain in Alzheimer's and other diseases."(177) How does this happen?

• One example is cigarette smoking, which can lead to neural death.

• Another is chronic untreated major depressive disorders, which are associated with loss of noradrenergic cells. (178)

• Cocaine habits create a crack (sort of speak) in the way the brain communicates! Cocaine causes white matter structural damage resulting in neurodegeneration. (179a)

Most long term pain medications have adverse effects on cognition, energy, moods, and increases our risk for stress and Leaky Gut Syndrome. (see pg 53)

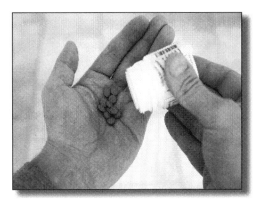

Medications That Drain The Brain

Montelukast, an asthma medication, may cause reactions including agitation, anxiety, depression, sleep disturbance, hallucinations, suicidal thinking, neuropathies (damaged nerves), and seizures. (80) This medication may not be suitable for long term use. Yet, most doctors don't openly explain the side-effects or change the medication protocol after 6 months of use. Sadly, studies reveal adult asthma increases our risk for dementia. (80a)

Sciatica nerve root pain and nerve root entrapment induce persistent mitochondrial disfunction. The use of anticonvulsants for neurogenic pain can be as common as epidural steroid injections. An abundance of opioids are commonly used for pain, as are muscle relaxants and non-steroidal anti-inflammatory drugs (NSAIDs). (81-82-83) All are linked to Alzheimer's!

NSAIDs may also cause significant GI damage, including Leaky Gut Syndrome. (84-85) All NSAIDs come with the risk of gastrointestinal ulceration. (86a)

➡ To be well, we must first pay attention to keeping our gut microbiomes healthy. (89) Bacteria factors and a functional blood-brain barrier is essential to maintaining central nervous system homeostasis. (85a)(86)

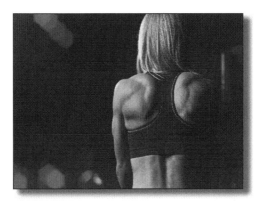

Spinal Decline & Alzheimer's

Poor spinal health plays an important role in Alzheimer's Disease. (167) This is because, postural deformities and cognitive functions are said to share a common pathophysiology. (168)

"A hallmark of age and neurodegeneration related cognitive decline is reduced neurogenesis!"(172) Endocrine Disrupting Chemicals have the potential to impair neurogenesis and cognitive function, and cause inflammation in both the developing and aging brain. (174) Environmental pollution can be found in poor spinal health and cognitive decline.

31

Neurodegenerative diseases comprise a condition in which
nerve cells, from the brain and spinal cord, are lost, leading to
either functional loss or sensory dysfunction (dementia). (173)
Additionally, researchers found a correlation between spinal
cord atrophy, Alzheimer's, and neurodegeneration. (111)
According to the Center for Neurodegenerative Disease
Research, "some spinal cords examined contained
neurofibrillary tangles," which is a marker of Alzheimer's
disease. (169)

Ankylosing spondylitis and dementia (Vascular and
Alzheimer's) have multiple causes and medical comorbidities
including obesity, depression and/or diabetes. Ankylosing
Spondylitis is a chronic inflammatory form of arthritis in the
spine. (170)

There are several medications used for Ankylosing
spondylitis.

One is Humira. Humira side-effects may include
gastrointestinal bleeding, jaundice, liver problems, painful
urination, poor vision, nerve problems, fungal infections, trouble
breathing, broken bones, confusion, and forgetfulness. "When
inflammation starts in (or is centered around) the gut, it can

affect our ability to absorb bone-building nutrients."(171) Glenn Frey, the founder of The Eagles, came to an untimely death in 2016 taking the prescribed medication Humira. He was 67 years old, suffering from Arthritis and Colitis.

➡It's critical to take care of gut health and bone health if we want to slow the progression of *Memory Stealers*. You can make an appointment with a holistic chiropractor for more information on how she/he can help keep your skeletal system aligned with exercise tips and adjustments.

Memory Stealers

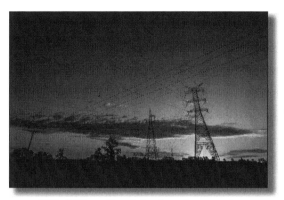

EMFs & Alzheimer's

Signs of overexposure to EMFs include muscle aches, insomnia, stress, and fatigue. But, that's not all, EMFs drain our brain!

The human body is a conductor of electricity. From atoms to organs, the human body depends upon its electrical systems to sustain life. We are life frequency in motion. Our nervous system is a 'hard-wired' network designed to carry sensory information and instructions, also in the form of electrical pulses.

In 1989 and 1990, a series of articles by Paul Brodeur in the New Yorker, entitled "*Annals of Radiation*: The Hazards of Electromagnetic Fields," shocked the nation into an awareness of the health dangers associated with these unseen energy fields."

Today, adults and teens are spending more and more time in schools (with exceptionally high EMF exposure) and on computer screens and cell phones. "Exposed students are complaining of headaches, difficulty concentrating, weakness, and heart palpitations, prompting their parents to take them to their family doctor or to their pediatric cardiologist to determine the nature of their problem."[46]

- Wireless radiation [40] can be linked to adverse biological effects on our DNA, [41] memory, sex hormones, [42] and the gut microbiome.

"Our planet has a rhythm that has played a major role in governing the evolution of life." Sending colluding signals to all microorganisms, Schumann Resonances drives the harmonizing pulse for life in our world. With the right kind of stimulus, we feel rhythm not only in the brain but in the body as well. This is the universal language of resonance." - Physicist: Winfried Schumann (47)

So, what happens when we don't have the right kind of stimulus? We end up with a sick brain.

➡ Our brain, high in frequency, is sensitive to the overuse of toxins, chemicals, and EMF pollution.

The Science on EMF Side-Effects

Thirst for domination & power increases planetary Alzheimer's

EMFs contribute to inflammatory conditions, poor gene expression, changes in the central nervous system nerve cells, and neurodegenerative diseases, stressing us to our core. (49)

1- Electromagnetic field exposure increases production of amyloid-beta, which eventually leads to Alzheimer's disease. (50) You do not have to be connected to the Internet to be exposed to the radiation generated by a wireless router. (51)

2- Studies support to the hypothesis that EMF exposure increases the risk of early-onset Alzheimer's disease. (52-53)

3- Wi-fi, smartphones, and EMF's have the ability to cause neurobehavioral disorders, which can disrupt blow flow. (54) The WHO's International Agency for Research on Cancer classifies EMF's as 'possible human carcinogens'. (55) EMFs can also interfere with the circadian system and damage the human liver. (56) EMFs can negatively influence hormones and increase the risk for depression.

39

4- Based on multiple studies, the Raines (1981) reports nineteen neuropsychiatric effects to be associated with occupational microwave/radiofrequency EMFs. (57)

5- "According to the Journal of Cerebral Blood Flow & Metabolism, EMFs from cell phones disrupt glucose levels."(58)

➡ It's time to question the obsessive-compulsive building of massive EMF towers all over the United States. As humans, we are undeniably about energy, rhythm, and frequency. (59) We communicate, hear, and respond to sound and energy through every pore of our body. EMFs can interfere with this communication.

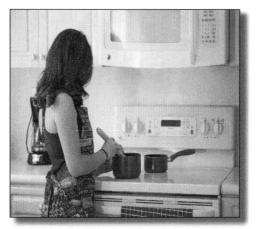

Oxidative Stress

"A consequence of neurodegenerative disease is severe mental and physical illness. ATP depletion and oxidative stress are thought to be the main mechanisms that cause all cell dysfunction."

"Oxidative stress emerges when an imbalance exists between free radical formation and the capability of cells to clear them."[60] Neurological diseases from oxidative stress include Alzheimer's, Parkinson's, multiple sclerosis, depression, and memory loss.

Studies show, there's a role of oxidative stress concerning major neurodegenerative disorders and blood flow. (61) Low blood flow can lead to imbalances in all mind and body functions. (62) "In fact, early-onset Alzheimer's shows issues involving arterial stiffness and blood-brain barrier dysfunction leading to hypoperfusion."(63) "Hypoperfusion is; disrupted perfusion of blood flow on brain structure and function."(64)

5 Avoidable Toxins

Chemical toxins play a role in oxidative stress

1. One is aluminum inside the pathological features of Alzheimer's. Consuming aluminum can be from cooking in aluminum pots and pans, some paints, salt as aluminum silicate, fluoride, and cosmetics. I've seen famous makeup artist use glues, wax prosthetics, paints, and sprays directly on the face of their models all in the name of beauty. An *illusion* where all can get disillusioned and deathly ill.

2. Opioid Use Disorder induces oxidative stress and increases addiction with little relief from inflammation. (87)

3. Moth Balls are a dangerous chemically made compounds that increase oxidative stress and DNA damage. (87a) Mothballs are solids that turn into a toxic gas. (87b) These adverse effects are felt in our brain, skin, and sinuses.

4. "The U.S. Food and Drug Administration has never approved any pigments for tattoos, and the inks are not actually developed for use in humans."(65) Can you imagine? These inks are found mostly in car paint or industrial pigments. And skin reactions to tattoos are not uncommon. (66) Tattoo inks cause oxidative stress and are cytotoxic, which means that they are toxic to our cells and can cause cell death! (67)

   According to Dr. Samuel Epstein, " As far as the brain is concerned, we have actual evidence of entry of tattoo ink into the brain producing toxic effects."(68)

   Inks can also contain hazardous polycyclic aromatic hydrocarbons (PAHs) and phthalates and are often contaminated with different microorganisms. (69-70) Exposures to persistent organic pollutants (POPs) PAHs and polychlorinated biphenyls (PCBs) have been found to be associated with neurological disorders. (71)

5. Synthetic & Artificial food color and dyes are chemical toxins. Artificial dyes derived from petroleum are found in thousands of foods. In particular, breakfast bars, candy, snacks, beverages, vitamins, and other products. (72) Artificial foods colors put our children at risk for brain drain! "The three most widely used dyes, Red 40, Yellow 5, and Yellow 6, are contaminated with known carcinogens. Even some fresh oranges are dipped in dye to brighten them and provide uniform color, says Michael Jacobson, executive director at CSPI." Another example is McDonald's strawberry sundaes, which are colored with Red 40. (72) Food dyes can be hidden in movie theater popcorn, store-bought cakes, salad dressing, snow cones, and Doritos. (73) Dyes cause neurobehavioral toxicity.

➡ Food colorants are linked to Alzheimer's Disease and learning difficulties. (73a-74a)

Oxidative Stress in Menopause

Chemicals can change genes on and off and disrupt brain function.

The female sex is one of the major risk factors for developing late-onset Alzheimer's disease. Studies show a woman's endogenous (disruptors inside our systems) and exogenous exposures (toxic exposures outside the body) during midlife and post-menopause influence Alzheimer risk.

"In 2011, researchers presented findings at a meeting of the Endocrine Society in Boston that revealed, women in their 40's and 50's who have extensive skin wrinkling are much more likely than their peers to have low bone mass. The problem is sugar. Studies show a chronic sugary habit accelerates bone loss at the spine and affects the efficiency in which the body metabolizes Vitamin D."[74]

Moreover, as with other organs, the premature aging of a woman's' skin is continuously exposed to multiple exogenous and endogenous stressors. [75] (I cover each stressor below) Premature aging is avoidable and menopause is not a death sentence. It's called '*change*' for a reason. The bottom line when we don't change we have an increased risk of Alzheimer's. How does this happen? Amyloid in the skin can induce protein aggregation in the brain. (76)

> When we look into the eyes of those who have Alzheimer's, we first see premature aging of the skin.

The good news is, it's possible that postmenopausal women who do not develop Alzheimer's or negative menopausal brain changes are attributed to healthy habits. These healthy habits include a diet consuming vegetables over refined sugary products, a healthy non-toxic skincare routine, and exercise in addition to intellectual stimulation.

➡Reading books is one form of intellectual stimulation.

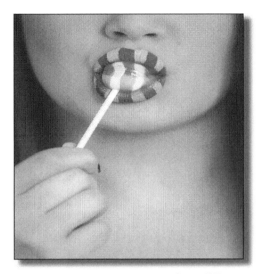

Accelerated Aging & AGEs

"When age is not a concern we never step away from the mirror long enough to look at our surroundings." CR

Alcoholism wreaks havoc in our body, causing advanced glycation end-products in our gut, liver, and brain cells. AGEs is the king of aging all organs simultaneously, and the queen of oxidative stress! In reading this book, so far, you'll find a tangled web of information acknowledging many relationships to *Memory Stealers* that begin with other disorders such as insomnia and obesity. You'll also find several common everyday habits that accelerate *Memory Stealers*, such as processed foods, sugars, and alcohol. Driving this home, I hope to show the connection between children and young adults suffering from adult diseases. Most are two-fold problems. If one suffers from depression, they may also have anxiety. If one has ASD, they may also have OCD.

The seriousness of 'stuck patterns' is what steals memories. Are you one that gives into your sweet tooth every night? The more *sugar and alcohol* we ingest, the more AGEs we produce. I've volunteered to help an elderly couple wash their floors and take out their trash once a week. Last week they had four large trash bags filled with empty bottles of alcohol.

Advanced Glycation End-products result from a domino effect set in motion anytime blood glucose increases. There is mounting evidence that suggests Advanced Glycation End-products caused by alcohol and/or processed sugary foods and can be implicated in the development of chronic degenerative diseases associated with Alzheimer's Disease, Cardiovascular disease, and Diabetes. (114-115)

Do you see the point? Truth be told, we're already witnessing early-onset dementia and Alzheimer's at a younger age.

In the last 60 years, food manufacturers and the processing of fast foods have contributed to advanced glycation end-products as flavor enhancers and colorants in foods to improve appearance, harming future generations to come. (116)

Ask yourself if you purchased any junk foods in the last 60 days? Please don't beat yourself up, we all do at one time or another. But why do we continue? It's all about the *illusion*? Everything in moderation is OK. But in reality, it's NOT.

The bottom line is Food Science is not only keeping our kids sick, tired and moody, the processed foods they eat adversely affects blood flow to their young brain harming gut microbes. Food Science targets children. How do we know this? Statistics found children eat more cookies, biscuits, chips, bread, cheese, peanut butter, and processed meats, than adults. (117)

Dr. Agnes Flöel said: "…even for people within the normal range of blood sugar, lowering their blood sugar levels could be a promising strategy for averting memory problems and cognitive decline as they age."

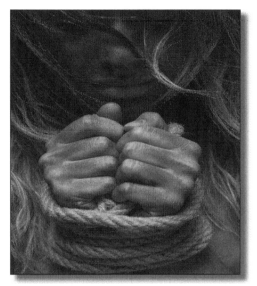

A Small Crack in Communication

There is crosstalk between all our systems, especially in times of inflammation. The skin sends feedback to the brain regarding stressors and can communicate with the central nervous system through hormones. (90-91) When inflamed, the skin-brain crosstalk may be implicated in skin rashes, psoriasis, and other skin disorders.

"Emerging evidence points to a bidirectional communication between the neuroendocrine system and gut microbiota." Communication can be disrupted by highly inflammatory habits, including consuming glutenous products. Gluten related products have a negative affect on good gut bacteria, our immune system, digestive system and nervous system, and therefore skin and brain cells can show unfavorable changes!

Sadly, gluten-free products, most times, only give us the *illusion* of health. We become disillusioned when we look at the label indicating all the other toxic ingredients that can compromise brain health.

"Research in psychoneuroimmunology and brain biochemistry informs us if we break communication pathways associated with nutritional intake, (with involvement in the central nervous system and immune function) this break influences an individual's psychological and physical health."(119)

Leaky Gut Syndrome is only one result of a break in communication. Its inflammatory nature presents itself in our gut, immune system and central nervous system. It's involved in Celiac disease where we may experience headaches, skin rashes, bloating, IBS, and joint issues first, before cognitive impairment, and neuropsychiatric disease.(120) A knee jerk reaction may be to first prescribe an anti-inflammatory medication for those symptoms.

If you already have Leaky Gut Syndrome, as I did, one may have multiple chemical sensitivities first. MSCs are the end result of a high toxic load as the nervous system becomes sensitized. (121) Multiple Chemical Sensitivities affects millions.

➡ Given the circumstance, when the body reacts to toxic exposures, it's better to see if you can remove the toxin first.

In Alzheimer's, we see the process of what I call 'inflamed communication.' Alzheimer's, metaphorically speaking, uses miles of beaded ropes called inflammation and slowly cuts off blood flow and oxygen trying to feed the central nervous system, gut microbiome, immune system, circulatory system, endocrine system, metabolic system, and the Endocannabinoid system. (92)

Memory Stealers

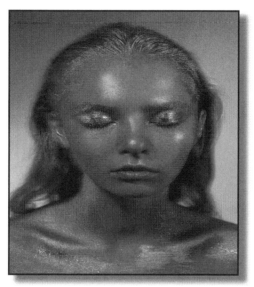

The Endocannabinoid System

The Endocannabinoid system is intertwined with our circadian rhythm and is an important regulator of intestinal function and the brain-gut axis. (93) The endocannabinoid system influences our metabolism, the central nervous system, the cardiovascular system, the respiratory system, the gastrointestinal system, the musculoskeletal system, and more. The job of the endocannabinoid system is to promote homeostasis!

"**Stress** is typically defined as any stimulus that represents a perceived or actual threat to homeostatic functioning." "Stress influences the immune system *and sleep patterns* through two routes; the hypothalamus–pituitary–adrenal axis and the autonomic nervous system. In the autonomic nervous system, poor sleep habits are associated with an increased incidence of cardiovascular disease."(97) Because circadian rhythms control hormone production, poor sleep habits can increase our risk for IBS, brain fog, lowered immunity, fatigue, and depressive symptoms. (98-99)

Physiological activity of the endocannabinoid system becomes deregulated during obesity and other related metabolic disorders. (94) Adding insult to injury, these disorders then increase our risk for Alzheimer's, causing accelerated atrophy in our brains' grey matter. (95-96)

Mercury stresses the endocannabinoid system and is a known neurotoxin. It has been shown that neurotoxins are dangerous to our brain, mouth, and other organs and tissues. Mercury disrupts our hypothalamic-pituitary-adrenal axis and can be found in fish, contact lens solution, old space heaters, and more. According to Dr. Blaylock, "flu vaccines contain mercury in the form of thimerosal."

➡There are never any safe levels of mercury exposure.

Pesticides such as chlorpyrifos and diazinon disrupt and alter normal eCB system function. Pesticides increase stress. The good news is we have studies suggesting that eating organic foods lacking pesticide residues may promote eCB homeostasis. (100)

Phthalates are plasticizers added to water bottles, tin cans, food packaging, and even the enteric coating of pharmaceutical pills. Phthalates may act as endocrine disruptors and/or carcinogens. They also block CB1. (101) "CB1 receptors are located in different areas of the brain, the immune system, and the heart."(102)

Plastics contain a variety of chemicals that impair hormone function. (102a) According to Paul Goettlich, plastics, their additives, and other processing chemicals are toxic at extremely low concentrations than at much higher concentrations. This is contrary to the FDA scientist's paradigm that, "The dose makes the poison," meaning that the higher the concentration, the more toxic something is."

We eat or drink things that are stored in plastic. So it's not hard to believe plastics are in our food. These plastics are called "Food Contact Substances" by the US Food and Drug Administration. (103)

We wear plastic clothing, we sit on plastic chairs, and so on, with the end result increasing our toxic load. We feel them in and on our skin, and so plastics are inside us.

We sleep on plastics. Flame-retardants, found in foam products, mattresses, furniture, and children's clothes, are found causal in neurological damage and growth retardation.

Our oceans eat plastic too! Unfortunately, we live in a sea of chemical exposures and while we absorb them they create *Memory Stealers*.

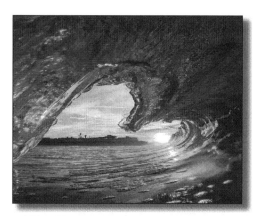

Getting To The Heart Of Alzheimer's

"Your heart tells you want you want and your brain makes it happen. If you constantly count your losses instead of what you are thankful for, you stand to loose both heart and mind."CR

Hypertension, HBP, heart disease, cholesterol imbalances, diabetes, obesity, fungal pathogens, stroke, gut microbiome, medications, and air pollution are interconnected with Alzheimer's Disease. All compromise the blood–brain barrier integrity and increase inflammation. (104)

The Brain-Heart Connection

▷ Air pollution is responsible for chronic alterations involved in vascular dementia and Alzheimer's. It's also found causal in cardiovascular disease. (104a) "In spite of the current standards, it is estimated that in the USA over one hundred million people live in areas that exceed recommended air quality levels." (105)

▷ Diabetes, a vascular disease, is intimately connected to heart disease and obesity, and compromises blood flow to the brain. Gut microbes can play a determining factor in diabetes. Unfortunately, if we don't address these connections we stand to lose millions more to diabetes by the year 2030.

▷ The use of the prescription Viagra, (sildenafil), for erectile dysfunction, is linked to the increase risk for myocardial infarction and may increase neurologic, emotional, or psychological disturbances and aggressive behaviors. (106a-b)

60

▷ According to journals.plos.org, anorexia can be seen as a microbial imbalance. Anorexia may begin with self-loathing. Left unattended, anorexia stresses the heart, snowballing to cardiovascular complications. "Anorexia is instrumental in poor oral health, and is disruptive in the hippocampal volume causing cognitive decline." Eating disorders, such as anorexia, keep us from absorbing nutrients from the foods we eat. "Anorexia also increases our risk for Leaky Gut Syndrome and central nervous system inflammation."(106-107-107a-108)

▷ Chronic cocaine-use is present in atherosclerosis. C-Reactive Protein is an inflammation marker that plays a key role in determining atherosclerosis and is linked to the development and progression of Alzheimer's. (109)

▷ Chronic inflammation is a hallmark in cardiovascular mortality."(46c)

▷ Stress disrupts all systems and organs without exception, leaving its ugly mark on our heart and brain. Stress, if we allow it, has the ability to increase our risk for *Memory*

Stealers, obesity, heart disease and depression. (110) The catch? Untreated 'stressful depression' affects more than 19% of the 35 million Elderly Americans. (110a)

▷ In 2013, the Journal of Tehran University Heart Center showed, "There're numerous unfavorable side-effects using antidepressants in the cardiovascular system including, bradycardia, hypertension, electrocardiogram (ECG) changes, electrolyte abnormalities and sudden cardiac death."(112)

➡In general, it's a lifetime of poor choices that makes us weaker, not stronger. "According to the WHO, eighty percent of heart attacks and strokes are preventable."(112a) What I find interesting is, the heart is a responsible organ. We need to know how to care for it *'responsibly'* before it stops taking care of us.

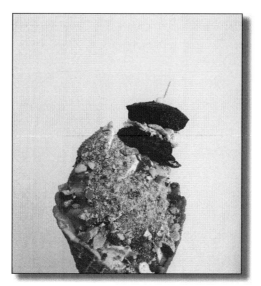

Stroke Protection

Most people I speak with are on 5 + medications a day, thinking they're healthy. What I hear half the time is, "I'm a potential stroke risk." I have to be very careful.

There are huge differences in being careful and having the ability to know how to add in self-care habits to your day.

You may receive a blood thinner medication and/or antidepressant, in order to be careful.

"Stroke is the second leading cause of death and the third leading cause of disability." And research revealed stroke is a major risk factor for Alzheimer's disease. (123) Taking Coumadin or other medications along with Coumadin (including aspirin or diuretics) may consequently change moods, gait, pain, appetite, taste buds, urine, and sleep habits for the worse. But, to some, these changes aren't important because they need the so-called no-stroke benefits of Coumadin.

"The main problem with the studies that show patients at risk of stroke, benefit from anticoagulation from Coumadin, is that they tested mostly high-risk patients on the typical (SAD) American Diet, not low-risk patients on a vegetable-plant-based diet. As one's diet changes to include more vegetation and fewer animal products and refined sugary foods, one's cholesterol comes into balance, one's blood pressure typically decreases, and one's risk of a heart attack or embolic stroke plummets."(124) With additional research, I've found foods also play a significant role in healing after we've suffered a stroke.

I have a friend on Coumadin that recently changed her diet to include more greens and less bread. She called me to ask why she couldn't stop her nosebleed. I told her to go see her doctor immediately. She did, and her doctor took her off this blood thinner.

➡It's about healing through the gut microbiome. Restoring health and balance to the gut microbiome decreases stroke risk. This information is key to understanding that 80% of strokes are preventable.

Memory Stealers

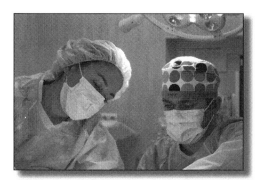

General Anesthesia & Cognitive Impairment

It seems doctors perform more surgeries in the last five to six years of our life. Anesthesia can be a hidden connection to long-lasting undesirable effects increasing inflammation, cognitive decline, and Alzheimer's disease. (126)

Clinical studies have also observed changes in cerebral spinal fluid levels of Ab and tau protein in patients following surgery with general anesthesia. (127)

Ketamine, an anesthetic, has been linked to the death of neurons and neuronal toxicity. And, believe it or not, is currently being investigated as an alternative treatment for depression. (128)

Another study was looking to discover whether heart surgery correlates with the development of cognitive dysfunction, which is a frequent complication of cardiac interventions. What they found is, "coronary artery bypass surgery provokes Alzheimer's disease-like changes in the cerebrospinal fluid."[129]

And, according to Anesthetics Pain Medicine and Intensive Care in London, cognitive impairment is very common in the elderly following general anesthesia used in surgery. [130]

➡ The sad news is, I've known many elderly people who have had an operation in the last 2 months of their life.

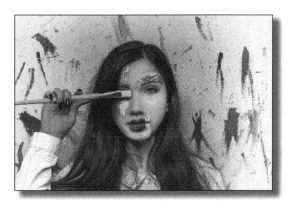

OTCs Can Steal Our Mind

"Every day you influence your universe through actions and thoughts. Your actions and thoughts are your energy field. Use them wisely."

I have a neighbor friend who frequently takes Benadryl and antacids along with NSAIDs, and washes them all down with ice-cold energy drinks. He almost cut his hand completely off when he started the chainsaw at work, last week!

Most times, a quick fix for a headache, flu, GERD, nausea, or constipation, is to take a pill and get back to your fast-paced life. If this has been your only solution for wellness, read on. Many medications taken by mouth can cause harmful side-effects damaging the endocrine system, brain, and gut microbiome.

Benadryl has been said to shrink brain size and cause cognitive impairment, along with constipation. (7-8) Because Benadryl disrupts hormones and good gut microbiome, and it increases our risk for dementia, Alzheimer's, and glioma.(9) Recreational use of antihistamines may be found causal in hallucinations. "Some second-generation antihistamines permeate into the brain tissue."(10) They can also increase appetite, disrupt the endocrine system, and B12 levels. In the end, they show similar attributes of a cocaine-like effect on the brain.(11)

Anticholinergics a group of medications for allergies, colds, depression, high blood pressure, and incontinence, may increase our increased risk of dementia. Why? Drugs such as those listed above along with antihistamines can block neurotransmitters! (12)

Antacids may create more indigestion problems. Copper and Vitamin B-12 deficiency may be caused by acid-suppressing drugs, including Prevacid and Prilosec. "Using antacids for heartburn and excess stomach acid may increase the risk of cognitive impairment in the elderly," according to a report in the

Journal of the American Geriatric Society. Antacids are taken to fight indigestion, but instead they diminish the enzymes needed to digest foods and nutrients critical to proper brain function. As crazy as it may sound, many antacids can contain lead, which can be linked to inflammatory issues and learning disabilities!

Cough Medicines adversely affect the central nervous system, may increase the risk for psychotic reactions, harms the respiratory system, and gut microbiome, causing stomach upset. Dextromethorphan, is an ingredient listed in cough medicine. A 2008 study found that "one in ten American teenagers has abused products containing DXM, making it more popular than cocaine, ecstasy, crystal meth, and LSD."[13]

"**MiraLax** is a laxative from Bayer Corporation made from polyethylene glycol 3350." Common side-effects of MiraLAX include psychiatric illnesses, nausea, abdominal cramping, bloating, and dizziness.[14-15-16]

Constipation can be a two-fold problem. Elimination is slow in transit time and a diet lacking necessary nutrients and fiber, cause dehydration, insomnia, and lack of exercise. A compromised gut microbiome changes for the worse when we are constipated for days leading to an unhealthy brain.

Dramamine is normally used for motion sickness.
Dramamine has also been abused by drug users, making it a
cheap and available high. It's an adenosine antagonist, which
can have negative side-effects on our heart, stress levels and
neurotransmitter functions. (17) Dramamine increases the risk of
an upset stomach and disrupts good gut microbes.

The gut microbiome is the ecosystem of bacteria that lives
within us. It is about 80% of our immune system. Microbes in
the gut microbiome don't just perform functions such as
digesting or synthesizing vitamins. They are connected with our
Central Nervous System and brain function. When disrupted, we
may experience hormonal imbalances, low serotonin levels, low
vitamin D levels, obesity, diabetes, dementia, and Alzheimer's.

➡It is safe to say that we may not need so many OTCs in our
medicine cabinets. Instead, I use non-toxic and anti-
inflammatory organic and wildcrafted essential oils. When we
use high-frequency essential oils these resonate with our own
body's frequency.

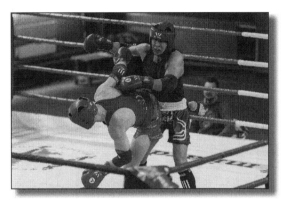

Brain Trauma

Both children and teens enjoy sports in high school and college. Some even as young as 16 are recruited to college campuses because of their ability to tackle their opponent fast, using extreme force.

A brain contact-sport can prove to be DISASTROUS for the future of a young brain. Muhammad Ali was just one example.

The hippocampus (where memories lie) is damaged with brain trauma. To prevent additional cracks in communication, we must prevent brain damage related to car accidents, physical abuse, and contact sports such as football and boxing.

➡Contact sports may cause irreversible harm to your child's brain. To slow, stop, or reverse the Alzheimer's epidemic, identification and reversal of causal factors must occur across our entire life."(122)

Chapter 2

The Injury To Our Senses

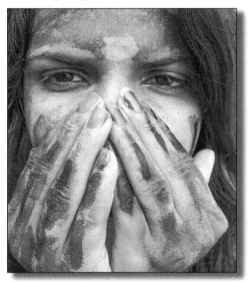

Damage Memories

"Living in the unconscious mind we rarely act or react to what is actually going on in front of our nose. The injury to our senses is real!" CR

Smell & Taste

The hippocampus is responsible for learning and emotional memories. It is located in our temporal lobe and part of the limbic system. And as such, memory-loss can begin with alterations and injury of the hippocampus.

Dying To Smell Good

The old saying goes, we choose our partners by how they smell, and we remember them this way! "The hippocampus and olfactory regions are anatomically close and both play a major role in memory formation."(132) Exposure to a single fragrance can contain a mixture of hundreds of chemicals creating imbalances in the brain and our endocrine system. Most of these chemically-made scents are not listed on the label. Household deadly scents are found in scented trash bags, bathroom cleaners, Swiffer's and more. Chemical sensitivities have been reported to develop within seconds of exposure. Just like exposures to cigarette smoke, toxic scents enter the body and bloodstream increasing our risk for oxidative stress causing free radical damage, premature aging, and poor mitochondrial health. (133) The end result is when damaged mitochondria is found causal in multiple diseases.

- The good news is according to Science Daily, "healthy mitochondria could stop Alzheimer's."(133a)

We absorb and breathe toxic chemicals on our clothes from laundry detergents which give rise to sinus infections, sore throats, brain fog, and poor cognitive function. We pore fluoridated and chemically created mouthwash in our mouth, get our car detailed using toxic chemicals, and overuse plug-in air fresheners. These first kill our tastebuds, our sense of smell, and then brain cells. The *illusion* is that we think we are going to somehow smell better, have our car smell better, or our homes smell better. We become disillusioned when these environmental pollutants take a choke hold on our lungs, liver, gut, and brain.

The nose is the portal of entry of airborne xenobiotics into the brain. (134) As a professional researcher and health/brain coach, I can say that olfactory loss can be the result from years of smelling, ingesting, and absorbing toxic exposures.(135)

"Research suggests Alzheimer's pathology could be mediated by environmental agents such as air pollutants that could reach the brain causing neuroinflammation." (136)

Amazingly, scientists have identified about 350 separate olfactory receptors in the human nose and also discovered about 150 of these receptors in other organs, including the heart and liver. (136a) Indeed, scent receptors are in nearly every human tissue. "Harm found in the olfactory bulb and tract is one of the earliest events in the degenerative process of the central nervous system in Alzheimer's."(137) Moreover, anosmia (loss of smell) can go unnoticed for many years before the diagnosis of Alzheimer's. (138) As delusional as it sounds, medical personal think its normal to have age-related decline in taste buds and loss of smell by the time we're 30 years old.

Neuropathy

Unbeknownst to most, we consume chemicals unaware of the damage these are doing to our hormones, sex life, metabolism, and immune system, compromising our brain function. "Neuropathic pain is a frequent manifestation of neurodegenerative diseases." (138a)

▷ *Processed foods, and refined sugars* can depress the immune system and other systems creating premature aging not only in our skin, but most importantly, the brain-gut axis causing neuropathy. How does this happen? Simple processed foods (frozen waffles, donuts, granola bars, and cereals) produce stress and anxiety damaging nerves creating a toxic internal environment slowing down the process of nutrients reaching cells.

▷ According to Researchers at UCLA, a diet steadily high in fructose from sugar beets and corn, slows down our brain, which can hamper memory and learning. The researchers discovered that genes in the brain could be damaged by fructose. This may impact memory and learning and could even lead to Alzheimer's disease. Aspartame is another toxin found in processed foods and drinks and has been implicated as one of the causes of neurodegenerative disease, inducing neurotoxic effects. (139) Toxins cause sensory nerve dysfunctions.

▷ *Smoking* damages our cell membranes in the brain, gut and skin. In fact, if children smoke between the age of 10 to 12, they can increase the risk for obesity and diabetes in their offspring. Smoking cigarettes, e-cigs and vaping not only accelerates the aging process, it decreases mitochondrial health and causes unfavorable changes in our skin's brain. These polluting habits decrease circulation throughout the body and therefore are linked to neuropathy, heart issues, and slow healing in our skin.

▷ *Malnutrition* can be linked to neuropathy by way of addictive substances or eating disorders and things that affect the GI tract causing low blood flow. Malnutrition, in this sense, is when our bellies are filled with junk, but we are not getting the necessary vitamins, nutrients and minerals we need to thrive. (140)

▷ Poor sleep habits are found in neuropathy. And while the hippocampus is vulnerable to sleep deprivation and chronic pain, "changes in hippocampal plasticity caused by painful stimuli may result in the development of neuropathic pain with cognitive decline as a side-effect."(141-142)

▷ Neuropathy could be attributed to drug intake including *antibiotics*, while prolong use of statins and alcohol abuse are among the causes of peripheral neuropathy. Blood pressure medications can also be found causal in Neuropathy. (143-144)

▷ Botox is a neurotoxin. "The Botulinum toxin is one of the most poisonous biological substances known."(145) Botox affects our thoughts and emotions. In 2018, multiple scientific studies were trying to prove the effectiveness of botulinum toxin, an injectable, for treating cramps in diabetic neuropathy. (146) In one study the Journal of Neuroscience authors wrote, "researchers injected the botulinum neurotoxin type A near the rats' whiskers. The toxin actually moved to the brain stem and appears to disrupt nerve cells' ability to communicate and may change spinal cord circuitry, the authors wrote." (147)

Botox injections can be dangerous to our health. Are you surprised?

Eye Health

What we may not realize is neurodegenerative diseases include ocular diseases (brain-eye connection) such as, macular degeneration and glaucoma. (157)

Dr. August Weismann, a German biologist, first introduced the wear and tear theory in 1882. He believed that the body and its cells were damaged by overuse and abuse. The organs, including the eye, are worn down by toxins in our diet and in the environment, by the excessive consumption of trans-fats, sugar, caffeine, alcohol, nicotine, and by the many other physical habits to which we subject our bodies. (148-149) This is cellular aging.

Researchers from Erasmus Medical Center in Rotterdam claim diet is related to the risk of developing macular degeneration. Those who ate worse-than-normal diets with low levels of nutrients actually had a 20 percent increased risk of disease. (150)

Inflammatory Ways We See The World

◆ Inflammation and stress are known to decrease circulation and found instrumental in macular degeneration. Not only does stress harm ocular health, it's influential in IBS, arthritis, diabetes, hypertension and more. (151) Inflammatory habits include but are not limited to a sedentary lifestyle, vaping, toxic exposures, and consuming low fiber sugary foods.

◆ Cataract and macular degeneration are increased by oxidative damage/oxidative stress which is causal in premature aging of all organs and tissues.

◆ Certain margarines and vegetable oils increase our risk for poor eye health. (152)

◆ High Blood Sugar levels increase ocular injury. Dietary sugars from sodas to teas, processed foods, crackers, and breads all disrupt our internal balance and play a causative role in poor eye health by way of obesity. (153-154)

◆ Poor Oral Microbiome is linked to poor eye health. "Oral bacteria in the upper quartile of the mouth were three times more likely to have glaucoma, suggesting a link between glaucomatous neurodegeneration and oral health." (155)

◆ Obesity harms eye health. The poor nutritional state of the retina has been consistently linked with adiposity. If one is overweight this increases our risk that macular degeneration will progress. (156)

Nutritional Factors for Eye Health

▷ We all need magnesium for optimal health. But most importantly, magnesium can protect the optic nerve and other ocular tissues from overstimulation. Some magnesium rich foods include, Asparagus, Spinach, Cashews, Almonds, Squash, Pumpkin Seeds, Figs and Kale. Magnesium may also assist in preventing obesity genes from expressing themselves. (158)

▷ Flavonoids are natural compounds found in vegetables, fruits, non-GMO organic olives, coconut oils and seeds. These help fight oxidative damage. (159)

▷ Chia seeds are omega-3 and consistently associated with decreased risk of Age-Related Macular Degeneration. (160)

▷ Get your sunshine before10:00 am for ocular wellness. (161)

▷ One of the essential nutrients needed to help prevent macular degeneration is lutein. Changes in lutein metabolism harms eye health. (162) Many vegetables contain lutein, but researchers found that most dark green, leafy vegetables contain a critical amount. I invite you to read *Nutrition, Diet, and The Eye.* (164)

▷ Carrots have the signature of the eye. Carrots have long been considered a food that helps us see in the dark. It appears, however, that the connection between your eyes and these nutritious veggies are well founded. The Department of Ophthalmology, at the University of Florida adds that macular degeneration can be largely prevented, and even reversed by eating more healthy fresh vegetables. (163) I juice my organic carrots with celery or add them to crunch up salads or dip them in homemade, organic hummus.

• The best supplement for eye health is water. Dehydration has detrimental effects on kidneys, eyes, cognition, and gut microbiome. [20] Pure clean filtered water is your best supplement for mind and gut health.

• The best way to take vitamins is to consume colorful fruits and veggies! A variety of colors from veggies every day will help meet our nutritional requirements. Prioritize Raw Foods First. You can chop up different organic vegetables for salads or soups each day and eat as many as you can prepared as many ways as you like.

Sound Impacts Memory

When memories fade so does sound!

Sound is energy and like all energies, can have a significant impact on our memory. Variations in air pressure travel across the room, into our ears, causing delicate sensors in our inner ear to move. Our inner ear converts this movement into electronic signals which are carried via neurons to our brain. Our brain identifies this information as birds, ocean waves, a violin, or conversations with friends.

Our brain generates frequencies called; *brain waves.*
For decades science has studied the human brain, mapping out which part controls our physiological functions and where our short and long-term memories are stored.

Specific frequencies can be in harmonic resonance or dissonance with our brain. Frequencies beyond our hearing range still have an impact on our cells. One example is, Ultrasound can help remove wrinkles and also see an unborn baby in the womb.

Environmental sound has a profound impact on our mood and our complex and delicate senses. Did we grow up in a loving home where our parents played classical music or a home with anger and constant conflicts?

Our facial bones resonate in unique frequencies called *formants*. The resonant frequencies of our facial bones are what make individual voices unique. Our facial bone structure impacts the clarity of our speech, enhances the fidelity of what we hear, and even how we think. If we are experiencing cognitive decline and premature aging of our bones, we can also be experiencing hearing loss.

A study from the National Institute of Arthritis and Musculoskeletal and Skin Diseases suggest potential links between declining cognitive function and a decrease in bone mass. (165)

As the digital world progresses, we're already witnessing hearing loss occur at younger ages. Constant sound bombardment and eating poor quality foods has been shown to have a significant long-term impact on our hearing, and while the exponential advances in technology provide a growing world of conveniences, the side-effects may result in future generations where *hearing loss* becomes the norm for society.

Do you seem less able to recognize sound? What disrupts hearing has a direct link to bone loss and osteoporosis. (166)

➡A beautiful quote I enjoy from *Louis Colaianni* is, "Sound speaks to the sensorium; the entire system of nerves that stimulates sensual response." What could be simpler then hearing beautiful music, thinking happy thoughts, and sharing loving emotions with someone you love. All these excite our senses while encouraging wellbeing.

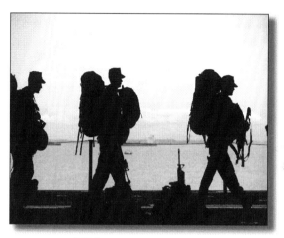

PTSD in Alzheimer's

"In the 1950s, the brain has been recognized as the center of the system controlling and regulating the physiological processes of the human body, and, currently we know the neuroendocrine and immune system networks are interconnected." (118) There are neuroendocrine aspects of PTSD. (118a)

"Evidence suggests that people suffering from post traumatic stress disorder have a higher risk for developing Alzheimer's disease." (179) Commonalities that affect both PTSD and Alzheimer's include multi-tiered and bi-directional crosstalk in inflammatory conditions, autoimmunity and major depression disorders. (178a-179)

Depression can be found in overwhelming feelings of anxiety, sleep depravation in the hippocampus, neurodegeneration, mental confusion, loss of interest in socializing, neurological issues, inflammation and gastrointestinal disorders. Sometimes PTSD can also co-occur in bipolar disorders (180) and in sexual abuse.

My aunt was abused during her childhood spent at a Catholic Orphanage.

The term PTSD wasn't coined back then. People just thought she suffered with mental illness (they called her crazy) and as she aged, it was labeled dementia. I believe, abuse can be intertwined with other disorders and it remains a whisper in the back of our minds for decades before it comes to a head.

Alzheimer's & PTSD Are Gut Related

As with any stress disorder, whether it be PTSD, Alzheimer's or others, we have to examine where the disconnection lies and bring frequency back into that area in order to regain health. This is where the gut microbiome can hold the key. (181) Science sees the gut microbiome as an organ. Unfavorable changes found in the gut microbiome create oxidative stress. (182-183)

Gut damage can occur with alcohol or substance abuse from people suffering from PTSD. (185) And, according to Scientific Reports, "exposures to heavy metal compounds have been shown to alter the diversity and composition of the gut microbiota."(184a)

According to the Department of Comparative Biomedical Sciences, "PTSD may not be solely a neurological pathology but involve multiple organ systems including the gut. (184) PTSD can be associated with Leaky Gut Syndrome because of an impaired gut barrier function.

This gives rise to leaky brain or leaky capillaries. Leaky capillaries is another term for neuroinflammation among alternative, integrative doctors. Arthur Toga, director of the USC Stevens Neuroimaging and Informatics Institute at the Keck

School of Medicine said, "If the blood-brain barrier is not working properly, then there is the potential for damage." "And, if the vessels aren't properly providing the nutrients and blood flow neurons need, we have the possibility of toxic proteins getting in."(185a)

➡Fermented Probiotic Foods are a good place to begin for improving good gut microbiome and brain function.

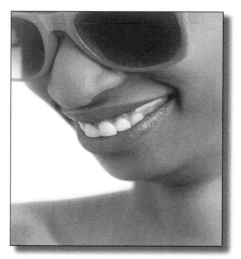

Periodontitis, PTSD & Alzheimer's

Mental illness has it's roots in the gut-brain axis and in the oral-gut axis (194)

Our teeth are instrumental in how well we age. The bones in our face, neck, mouth, and ears work in harmony with each other. This is how we communicate, sing, think, and chew. As we get older, poor oral health may cause us to loose teeth which could definitely affect memory loss. Chronic stress, depression and anxiety can significantly enhance the pathological progression of periodontitis." It involves the hypothalamic-pituitary-adrenal axis as a result of emotional pressure suffered for a prolonged period, over which an individual perceives they have no control."[25] Stress may prevent us from paying attention to good oral health. In 2014 Research suggests that several types of spirochetes bacteria, including periodontal pathogens, may be involved in the pathogenesis of Alzheimer's with a probable causal relationship. [201]

According to the Department of Prosthodontics, School of Dental Medicine, Rijeka, Croatia, "PTSD patients had more TMD diagnoses." [202a]

A major 2019 study in *the Journal of Oral Microbiology* discovered that bacterial populations from the mouth make their way to the gut microbiota. Poor oral bacteria can alter immune responses and potentially lead to systemic diseases. [202]

Toxins can change oral microbiome. Teflon/Dupont electric toothbrushes contain endocrine disrupting toxins. The dangerous chemicals that make up Teflon prevents our immune system from fighting off infections which means Teflon plays a significant role in inflammatory illnesses. [196]

• PTSD and tooth loss can negatively influence cognitive function in various ways, one of which is inflammation induced by periodontal disease. Periodontitis is linked to the inflammatory process affecting the bloodstream and the brain contributing to cognitive decline. (195)

• Chronic periodontitis, with amalgam fillings shows a slightly higher likelihood of Alzheimer's disease. (197-200)

• Chronic fluorosis, apart from affecting the skeleton and teeth, has significant adverse effects on the brain, metabolic function, gastrointestinal function and endocrine function. (203) The bottom line, fluoride exposure is connected to Alzheimer's, and poor dental hygiene is linked to brain degeneration. (204-205)

Memory Stealers

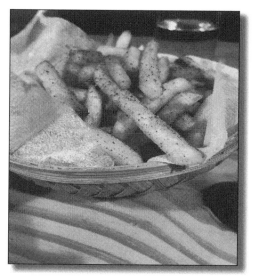

Path to Neurodegeneration

A Fat to Forget!

Poor choices of fats can be found in fried chicken, french fries, fried shrimp, donuts, cookies, apple pie, pancakes, frostings, powdered creamers, and more causing neurodegeneration. It's not about everything in moderation. Even moderate intake of trans-fats increased our risk for Alzheimer's Disease.

Trans-fats harm our central nervous system and brain, causing significant adverse changes in mood and mitochondrial health. Trans-fats have an association with increased aggression, diabetes, obesity, and premature skin aging. (206-207) Trans-Fats scar brain tissue, harm arterial cells and cardiac health, increases insulin resistance and causes aggression leaving us depleted of energy and memory. (208-209-210)

Soybean Oil

Soybean oil is found mostly in processed foods, livestock feed, and restaurants and has been found causal in inflammation, obesity and diabetes paving the way for neurodegeneration. (211) In 2014 studies revealed, "soy consumption may be a significant contributor to Alzheimer's dementia, and it cannot be excluded as a possible contributing cause." (212)

Sugar

Sugar can increase our risk for neurodegeneration. "High-sugar diets promote weight gain and insulin resistance predisposing us to type 2 diabetes.(213) So it's no surprise that diabetes is a risk factor for Alzheimer's.

Not only does sugar keep us sick, overweight, toxic, and depressed, "the cultivation and processing of sugar produces environmental impacts." This happens through the loss of natural habitats, intensive use of water, heavy use of agro-chemicals, discharge and runoff of polluted effluent and air pollution."(214)

Glyphosate

Glyphosate along with a western diet has the ability to induce diseases such as depression, and obesity.(186-187) Yet another study cites, "Glyphosate is considered highly toxic causing gastrointestinal disorders, diabetes, autism, and Alzheimer's."(193) "Glyphosate damages all cellular systems throughout the body, causing inflammation and oxidative stress."(188) Researchers even suggest glyphosate significantly alters the central nervous system. (189) Recently, the World Health Organization has just come out with a position that glyphosate is a level 2 "probable carcinogen". (192)

Many epidemiological studies have described adolescent-related psychiatric illness and sensorimotor deficits after exposure to a Glyphosate based herbicide.(190) Why? Glyphosate is an endocrine disruptor and endocrine disruptors, as a class, have an interesting property that very low doses are far more toxic to our health than higher doses. Glyphosate prevents the detoxification of glutamate by glutamine synthase.(191) Pesticide residue is found in monosodium glutamate. (191a) To make matters worse, MSG *neurotoxicity* increases beta amyloid plaque in animal hippocampus. (131) MSG negatively influences our taste buds, eating behavior, increases risk for obesity and oxidative stress. It's found in canned soups, salad dressings, drinks, breads, Chinese foods, natural flavors, some dairy products, and more. Most times it goes unlisted.

Noteworthy. Natural and artificial flavors are not natural and not found in nature.

Do you love French fries? You can cut your own organic sweet potatoes and bake them at home. Same goes for pizza, using fresh ingredients such as organic nut cheese, fresh basil, herbs and tomato and lay them on a freshly-made cauliflower crust. Replace your favorite soda with some fresh squeezed lemon in some sparkling water. When we make simple changes in daily habits, we can look forward to eliminating early dementia and Gut Dysbiosis, by modifying the gut microbiome. This is where we combat neurodegeneration. (215)

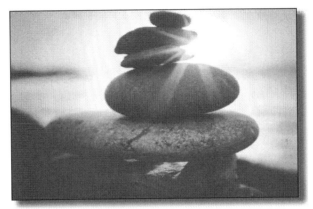

Take Back Your Mental Health

"Stress, toxins, and a poor diet, are counter productive to brain, gut, and our overall wellness." CR

I- Be Sun Smart

Allow the body and mind to communicate via sunlight.

"When our internal clock is not accord with the cycle of the Sun, the inconsistency induces helplessness at day time and leads to symptoms of insomnia at night." Adequate sunlight improves digestion, reduces brain fatigue, depression, boost neurotransmitters, immunity, and vitamin D supply. (216-217)

Early morning 'sun salutation' is sun-smart. There are benefits when ingesting vitamin D through sunshine. "When vitamin D3 is produced in the skin, 100% of it is potentially bound to the vitamin D binding protein.

When vitamin D3 is supplemented, 40% is lost." (218)

2- Crack The Code For Obesity

Remove mold and toxic chemicals that can cause indoor air pollution. A study published in the Office of Integrative Medicine shows that GMOs are contributing factors to the obesity epidemic. (219-220) If we rethink what food really is, it is energy. The energy of our food becomes our mind. Foods that are dead, processed, altered, highly salted, or toxic, are low to zero energy sources allowing inflammation and weight gain to creep in.

I believe our tummy feels so much better when we avoid wheat and corn grains. Why? Because these highly processed simple carbs are treated with inflammatory chemicals, pesticides, and hormones to increase shelf-life and your bottom line, belly fat! The result is glue in the gut and sugar in the blood. Regardless of any genetic predisposition, it's possible to reduce obesity and increase brain and body health by reducing our toxic load.

3- Take care of neurotransmitters in the gut

Our nervous system and our immune system are not independent systems but are closely associated and use the same makeup of neurotransmitters. (223) A healthy gut, for instance, is necessary for healthy neurotransmitters. Scientists have found gut bacteria produce neurotransmitters such as serotonin, dopamine, and GABA and play a key role in mood and mental health. (226) When levels of neurotransmitters in the brain adversely change its attributed to inflammatory conditions in the gut. Furthermore, when we least expect it, digestive, metabolic, and central nervous system disorders happen first before Alzheimer's. (225) Why do we need to be concerned? Mental illness is an inflammatory condition. (224) "The gut microbiota has a connection in depression, stress, and autoimmune diseases of the Central Nervous System."(125) Unfortunately, according to Johnson and Johnson Pharmaceutical, Research and

Development, Drug Discovery, autoimmunity-induced cell death is found in Alzheimer's. (225a) When we take care of our gut, we take care of our brain. Moreover, when we take care of neurotransmitters, we take care of immunity at the same time.

In 2012 studies showed insomnia might be a result of the decrease of GABA. (227) This information is significant, as suffering from chronic insomnia has a hidden connection for psychiatric problems.

4- Exercise

The brain and gastrointestinal tract work better together when we exercise. Personally, I love walking about 5 miles a day. Exercise helps me work smarter and sleep sounder. What I have found is, daily exercise is the best prevention for Alzheimer's.

Want new brain cells, EXERCISE! (228) Without exercise, the lymphatic system, lungs, digestive system, brain cells, and emotional health becomes stagnated.

5- Be Product Wise

Check the products in your home environment such as fragrances found in cleaning products, body lotions, shampoos, conditioners, candles, and the list goes on. You may discover that these products are produced from chemicals. Some of us may experience the effects of multiple chemical sensitivities sooner than others. However, it is abundantly clear that most illness in people and pets are triggered by toxins in, on and around us. You can find and purchase non-toxic organic products instead.

6- Increase Magnesium

Recent evidence suggests that low levels of Magnesium were implicated in the pathogenesis of Alzheimer's. [229] Diuretics, Antacids, Birth Control Pills, Chemotherapy, Tetracycline, Blood Thinners, and Corticoids, are just a handful of medications that can lead to magnesium loss. Foods that contain healthy levels of magnesium include, but are not limited to, organic spinach, watermelon, broccoli, raw almonds, lentils, and pumpkin seeds. Multiple studies suggest that increasing brain magnesium levels leads to the enhancement and improvement of memory function. [230]

7- Consume Antioxidants

Beets are a powerful antioxidant. (231) They help prevent dementia and improve cognitive function, high blood pressure, vascular function, insulin resistance, cancer, and inflammation! Wow, that's a mouthful!

Turmeric is an antioxidant and has been found to reduce amyloid plaque buildup. It helps to prevent cognitive decline and brain cells from stroke damage, and promotes the growth of new brain cells!

Antioxidants from whole foods have been found helpful in fighting oxidative stress. (232) Adding in foods rich in antioxidants and avoiding junk foods can be instrumental in the prevention or reduction of high anxiety disorders. (233) But, even more importantly, studies reveal that antioxidants are an essential part of prevention in the pathological process of Alzheimer's. (234)

Glutathione is a powerful antioxidant and detoxifier. Our bodies need glutathione for detoxification pathways to work correctly, to flush out toxins, pollutants, and heavy metals. In other words, glutathione supports our immune system.

"Glutathione in the epithelial lining fluid of the lower respiratory tract is thought to be the first line of defense against oxidative stress."(235) "Glutathione supports our mitochondria and reduces our risk of Parkinson's and Alzheimer's Disease." (236-237)

Asparagus contains more glutathione than most other vegetables. I love asparagus and highly recommend them for inflammatory conditions, including Alzheimer's, RA, and children with autism and ADD. Other foods that raise glutathione levels are broccoli, Brussels Sprouts, cabbage, cauliflower, avocados, peaches, and watermelon. Several spices raise glutathione levels, including organic cinnamon, and cardamom. Alpha Lipoic Acid (ALA) promotes the synthesis of glutathione in the body. Food sources of ALA include spinach, broccoli, tomatoes, peas, and Brussels sprouts. When your grandmother said, eat your broccoli she knew broccoli can stimulate brain regeneration.

➡The good news is, when we consume foods that boost antioxidant activity, we assist the body in *purging toxins*.

8- Add-In Good Fats

A shortlist of Brain-Boosting fats includes organic avocados and raw organic walnuts.

9- A Work In Progress

There is a way out from chronic stress. The daily practice of meditation also helps reduce stress and cellular aging! (238) According to Dr. Epstein, "There is an ever-growing body of evidence pointing to the role of the mind and its healing power in the treatment of stress, pain, mental, emotional, and physical illness. Meditation changes gene expression, while acupuncture, yoga, and visualization are alternative modalities for stress-related disorders." (239-240)

10- Play Music

Music is a universal language that lives deep within our spirit and influences our soul. Musical vibrations and frequency can bring about tranquility and relaxation. Humans and Mother Earth respond positively to awesome sounds. Soft relaxing music can even help us fall asleep at night. Music touches people's hearts and can resonate calm and healing in all organs.

11- Microbiome Connection & Relationships!

The brain-gut axis is intimately connected and works in tandem in everything we do. This team determines decision-making skills, emotions, how we work through stress, and how well we relate with others. Moreover, this brings me to talk about how we choose our mate by their gut microbiome connections.

Yes, it's true! We make intimate gut to gut connections. But first we kiss mouth to mouth. Together our lips share microbes. Our lips and mouth have a direct connection to our intestines and our immune system! This innate ability is key to lasting relationships. If you have a healthy microbiome, and your date is an alcoholic or smoker, you are less likely to continue the relationship for the long term. If you consistently eat junk foods and your partner eats junk foods, you may be a match, but not necessarily a good one.

The body contains trillions of bacteria and other microorganisms that inhabit all our surfaces; skin, mouth, sexual organs, and especially our intestines.

Diet and Lifestyle are not only critical for the health of our brain, immune system, endocrine system, and the metabolic system; they are critical for healthy long term relationships!

Noteworthy. Our brain can steadily deteriorate from toxic lifestyle habits. What's fascinating is, "Cambridge scientists have, for the first time, created cerebral cortex cells! These cells make up the brain's gray matter from a small sample of human skin." The researchers' findings, which were funded by Alzheimer's Research UK and the Wellcome Trust, were published in Nature Neuroscience. (241a)

Chapter 3

Psychobiotics

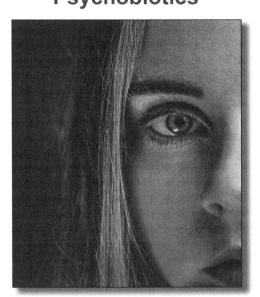

A Trendy Frontier

Eighty Percent of teenage girls are on a diet and moody. Fifty Percent have fatigue. Seventy Five percent have digestive issues. There is over a four hundred percent increase in prescribed antidepressants.

Psychobiotics

While not likely recommended by naturopathic or practicing holistic doctors, Big Pharma is touting Psychobiotics as a new frontier in neuroscience and possibly even the next generation of treatment for mental illness. There are several reasons why Psychobiotics can be a dangerous practice.

In today's society, addictive behaviors, gastrointestinal stress, oxidative stress, environmental stress, emotional stress, a sedentary lifestyle, pollution, and sleep deprivation are all typical traits adding to the development of obesity, Alzheimer's, anxiety, and mental illness.

Numerous studies have shown that psychological stressors suppress beneficial bacteria and elevated blood glucose levels, increasing our risk for insulin resistance. The point is that insulin resistance is just one of many disorders associated with cognitive decline and mood changes. (1)

Presently, we live in a world where stress-induced changes to our gut microbiome negatively affects cognitive function and increase our risk for *Memory Stealers*.

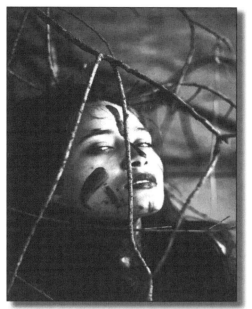

Why Hormones Matter

The Gut Microbiome is described as a neglected endocrine organ!

Male and female hormones affect our gut microbes, and brain structure, which plays a role in hormonal imbalances. The Journal of Clinical Endocrinology & Metabolism describes adipose tissue as a complex, essential, and highly active endocrine organ and plays a role in energy metabolism. (1a)

Gut microbes are in charge of cognition and emotions, including depression. Moreover, our liver and gut microbiome closely interact and are altered by diet. (2) What we put in our gut sparks brain cells, skin cells, emotions, our immune system, hormones, and electrical activity. (3)

Unbeknownst to most, endocrine disruption is one of the most prominent causes of mental instability, causal in part by pollution, toxic exposures, and medications with conventional foods at the top of that list. You'll see me talk about endocrine disruption throughout my book because it's significant in *Memory Stealers*!

High concentrations of indoor pollutants (endocrine disruptors) have never been tested for safety. These decrease the body's electrical activity and can be responsible for hormone imbalances, emotional imbalances, (anxiety and mood disorders) blood sugar imbalances, obesity, and neurodegeneration.

Over the years, I've seen abusive habits become lifestyle habits paving the way for the increasing rate of mental instability. We may be manipulated into thinking junk foods are the fuel of the future, *OR* we cannot live without our beloved scents from air fresheners and dryer sheets, *OR* a thirteen-year-old child needs birth control. The results are changing the way a child goes through puberty. These changes puts children at risk for mental instabilities.

Children today suffer from diabetes, herpes, obesity, depression, anxiety, HBP, Gerd, & Cancer. Medications include, but are not limited to, Statins, Beta Blockers, Tagamet, Famciclovir, Zantac, PPIs, Antidepressants, and more.

Beta blockers' side-effects may include depression, insomnia, and fatigue. Statins increase insomnia and show unfavorable changes in blood sugar levels, weight, and gut microbes. Side-effects from antidepressants include insomnia, poor gut microbes, depression, and increased risk for suicide.

Studies found a hidden connection between poor immune function and a damaged gut microbiome where schizophrenia, ASD, and depression are located. (5) If we look at types of medications prescribed for these behavioral disorders, we'll find them in the benzodiazepine or antipsychotics family. Antipsychotics, commonly prescribed for children and adolescents negatively affect the gut microbiome, metabolism, promote antibiotic resistance, and add to the obesity epidemic.
(6-7)

➡When we put an end to inflammatory factors that influence and adversely change our hormones, we then put an end to the way we pollute our universe, our brain, our gut and then we may decrease our risk for mental illnesses. (4)

100 Years Spent Improving the Gut

In **2014** researchers discovered, "there are essential gut microbes involved in endocrine regulation, and it's possible to use probiotics to treat or prevent metabolic syndrome and stress-related disorders."(8)

In **2015** studies found "The Gut-Brain Axis is the missing link in depression."(9)

In **2015** my book, *Path to a Healthy Mind & Body,* you may discover a *clean way* of living in a toxic world. (10)

In **2019** we made progress according to new research that's found Cannabidiol, a non-psychoactive chemical compound, has the ability to decrease anxiety. (11) Furthermore, Cannabidiol has anti-inflammatory effects and is similar to that of established antibiotics.

It was 100+ years ago the term "probiotics" was introduced. Recently, medical professionals agree, "manipulating the microbiota, either by prebiotics, probiotics or fecal microbial transplantation, seems rationale for the prevention and treatment of disease."(12) This is where interest in probiotics began. (13)

For about the last 28 years, we've been improving gut microbiota and anxiety on our own with the use of probiotics, prebiotics, colloidal silver, and fermented foods such as fermented sauerkraut and kimchi. (14) Probiotics are not chemicals. (15) Probiotics are live microbes that produce a health benefit that involves building immunity.

Most of my clients enjoy non-prescription probiotics from fermented non-dairy food sources. These have a positive influence on the intestinal microbiota and gut-brain communication. For instance, "*Lactobacillus pentosus* from fermented cabbage (kimchi) can improve mental functioning and hippocampal production."(16) I also discuss implementing calming *Me-Time* ways to handle anxiety. Choices include deep breathing exercises, meditation, jogging, massage therapy, diffusing organic essential oils, drinking calming herbal teas, yoga, and reading before bed.

Nevertheless, lately, there's talk about a new kid on the block. Psychobiotics! Studies suggest Psychobiotics are in the pursuit of happiness, as their job will be to improve microbiome and mental diseases at the same time. (17) Ask your doctor if it's right for you. "It's called disease mongering. (18) The effort to sell pharmaceuticals based on the creation of perceived need, a term introduced by health-science writer Lynn Payer in her book: *Disease-Mongers: How Doctors, Drug Companies, and Insurers Are Making You Feel Sick.*

In U.S. news reports, there's a different perspective on defining what our children need. Children and young adults are suffering from shyness, social phobias, hormonal changes, and anxiety causing mood changes, and they NEED to be medicated. There's a Buzz we are experiencing, an excitement if you will, about how Big Pharma can use Psychobiotics on our children for all phobias and mood problems. (19)

There may be grave holes in this theory!

- Anxiety disorders, though sharing some commonalities with depression is a different mental illness. (20)

- "When a condition like social phobia becomes a marketing "fig leaf" for a pharmaceutical company, we all lose because the results of clinical trials get sealed, left unpublished and inaccessible, the names of leading figures in the profession get put on ghost-written articles, and a dependence on pharmaceutical company funding develops. (21) The renaming of social phobia as social anxiety disorder is symbolic of what can happen."

- What I understand to be true is, social phobia is not the same as social anxiety *AND* antidepressants can add to the development of more anxiety disorders.

- In 2016, social phobia was described as anxious in social situations, fear in performance situations, and alike. (22) The National Health Service from the UK describes Social

Anxiety/Social Phobia as a long-lasting and overwhelming fear of social situations. (23)

However, fear, worry, and self-consciousness do not make a disease. Humans love connecting with others. We are social animals.

Most of us have had to deal with anxiety and fear more than a few times in our lifetime. Our youth today have a challenging future ahead of them with outstanding musical technology, iPhone technology, AI technology, and electric car technology.

Forty years ago and it still holds true today, teens act out like jokesters, bright and bold, in front of classmates. They can even enjoy working at a job after school. Kids can be outgoing and love to be seen, or some are shy and enjoy watching what others do. Shyness can come from inherited traits, learned from role models, or life events. There is never one size fits all. However, shyness has never been labeled a disease, until now.

Noteworthy, I do agree fears and anxiety can occur when girls are forced to share bathrooms with boys, and just possibly, there is too much time spent on cell phones, violent video games, or television, which can and will inhibit social abilities.

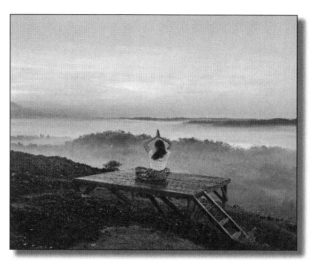

The Emotional Mind

Rupert Sheldrake, PhD, a biologist and author said; "Where are our minds located? We have been brought up to believe that they are inside our heads, that mental activity is nothing but brain activity. Instead, I suggest that our minds extend far beyond our brains; they stretch out through fields that link us to our environment and to each other. As soon as we accept the theory that the mind is more extensive than the brain, a whole range of unexplained phenomena begin to make sense... These include the sense of being stared at."

Kids consistently test parents to see if they can win an argument or two. In reality, kids learn from how a parent responds to their emotional outburst. Sometimes, emotions make no rational sense at all, but they are necessary for life. It is natural biological wiring.

Emotional intelligence means we have the ability to manage and recognize our emotions. The concept of emotional intelligence is self-awareness. How do we do this? From day one, we learn about nurturing habits, self-esteem, and social skills from the people who love us most, and others as we connect and relate with the universe around us. In children, higher emotional intelligence is positively correlated with better social relation skills and better psychological well-being as well. (24)

There are also differences in the social mind. It's called social intelligence. It's where we know how to recognize cues and social rules when relating to others. Being socially intelligent makes us good listeners, and then we are better able to converse and feel comfortable on several subjects of interest. Where emotional intelligence and social intelligence meet is understanding emotions!

➡It may be safe to say; there are differences in the emotional and social mind rather than calling differences a disease.

Mental Health First-Aid

Big Pharma uses the argument, "In a dysfunctional gut flora, disease can occur." This is true. However, may I add, in the U.S., we have a structured system designed to keep people sick and dependent on drug treatments, never curing or eradicating the root cause of their disease.

Anyone can relate to the fact that a dysfunctional gut flora can be linked to poor eating habits, chronic stress, and environmental toxins. And, fast-food science has, in retrospect, undermined the health of our gut microbiome and, therefore, our brain, for the last 60+ years. So why do we need Psychobiotics now? Fear! Fear-based thinking is, 'we need Big Pharma to fix all ailments.' And children are their latest fear-based experiment.

I call it Double Vision! A Big Pharma slippery slope leading back to their vision they have for our children. Children are suffering from shyness, social phobias, and anxiety they say, and they *need* intervention. Drugs!

Time and time again, we see the powers that be, using medications as social control.

My arguments against over-medication include one day, a child can feel confident and the next day, feel overwhelmed and insecure because they are experiencing hormonal changes. It's very normal when you're young. One week a child may be paralyzed with fear because they are expected to give a speech in front of the class, and the next day, he may perform like a math wizard with 40 students watching in amazement! There are science projects that some children enjoy while others can't stand the sight of.

Other fears can be from computer technology. Sharing emails/ text on a computer can become extremely impersonal or even destructive when written, because we're not looking directly in the eyes of the receiver, giving rise to social phobias. Granted, children are confined in a classroom more than we were years ago and have been put in dangerous situations when shootings occur. But, never do we see Pharmaceutical Companies taking the blame for the drugging of our children in such cases. What caused those mental breakdowns in teens is conveniently avoided.

➡️More often than not, we need to offer a drug-less option for social fears. I believe if we were to teach children powerful modalities to recognize and tame stress we can help them create individual/personalized go-to remedies for anxiety issues. From this one step, we would see fewer opportunities for children to grow into stressed and drugged adults, with poor decision-making skills.

As Big Pharma grows larger, children are getting sicker. It's an unfortunate situation for all.

"Researchers discovered that children in the United States are not only prescribed medications at a high rate; they are also increasingly being prescribed medicine to address "off-label" ailments. [25] An example of this would be taking antidepressants to treat symptoms of ADHD. Plus, many drugs prescribed for children have not been rigorously tested in children, according to the Food and Drug Administration." [26] I believe the FDA is supposed to protect consumers from harm.

In **2008** the National Institute of Mental Health was given the grant to study the effectiveness of the abortion drug 'mifepristone' as an antidepressant. (27-28-29) It's not a coincidence that "NIMH is the largest research organization in the world, and is specializing in mental illness."(30)

In **2013** studies from UCLA suggest the drug scopolamine is good for social phobias and anxiety disorders. (31) The side-effects of this drug include constipation, difficulty breathing, confusion, and paranoia, among others. (32) ClinicalTrials.gov used scopolamine in their studies for anxiety and social phobias. They also used Paroxetine, an antidepressant, with side-effects that include racing thoughts, confusion, tremors, and unusual internal bleeding. (33) Again in recent clinical trials, the drug JNJ-42165279 was tested to improve symptoms of Autism Spectrum Disorder, as well as phobias and anxiety disorders. (34) It's developed by Janssen Pharmaceutica and owned by Johnson & Johnson. (35) In clinical trials, it left one volunteer dead. (36)

In 2018 the National Institute of Health funded the science that supports new drugs. From the NIH website, I found social anxiety is more than just shyness. (37) And then, the NIH talks about the benefits of benzodiazepines being effective in relieving anxiety. (38)

Dr. Kelly Brogan asked, "what happens when we let drug companies tell doctors what science is? (39) We have an industry and a profession working together to maintain a house of cards theory in the face of contradictory evidence." (40)

Memory Stealers

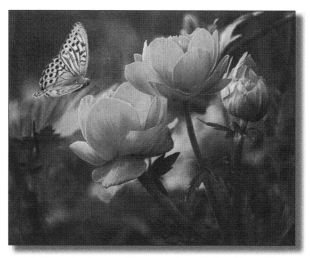

What Are Psychobiotics?

It looks like about ten years of study to come up with the term Psychobiotics. I found the search for commingling Tetracycline with probiotics began back in 2007. (41) In this study, researchers define Psychobiotics as a living organism that, when ingested, produces a health benefit in patients suffering from mental illnesses. (42) *Here, adequate amounts of probiotics are undefined.*

Psychobiotics, an emerging probiotic in psychiatric practice! (43) Psychobiotics will be used for the effective management of various psychiatric disorders. (43) *Here, I would like to see more strategy and clarity.* Psychobiotics will include, antibiotics which may include tetracycline, antipsychotics, antidepressants, prebiotics, and some form of probiotics, which they haven't decided on yet! (44-45) Some studies suggest Prozac can act as an antibiotic. (46-47) What they do not say is, Gingerol or garlic are natural antibiotics. (48)

Both antibiotics and antipsychotics may also be classified as Psychobiotics. (49) Antipsychotics are linked to brain shrinkage as well as killing brain cells. Psychobiotics will include drugs such as antidepressants and antipsychotics for changing mood, appetite, and sleep issues. (50)

The sad news is, "Psychotropic medications can contribute to the emergence or aggravation of physical diseases and weight gain." (51) Science concurs, "Psychobiotics still need to be tested in the general population, with the objective to reduce doses of psychotropics."(52) Pushing ahead, researchers believe, "a range of conceptual and technical issues require exploration, which will provide further mechanistic insights and pave the way for the emergence of systematic and efficient Psychobiotics."(53)

According to The WHO

▷ According to the WHO, probiotics are defined as "Live
microorganisms administered in adequate amounts." (this
study was done with milk powder and live lactic acid
bacteria.) Lactic acid bacteria (LAB) are Gram-positive,
non-spore forming cocci, coccobacilli, or rods, which
generally have non-respiratory (fermentative) metabolism
and lack true catalase." (53a)

▷ "The latter anxiolytic effect has even led to the emergence
of the new term, Psychobiotics, coined by Dinan as a "live
organism that, when ingested in adequate amounts,
produces a health benefit in patients suffering from
psychiatric illness." (54-55)

▷ Studies later proved *L. rhamnosus* might not be a beneficial
probiotic.(56) Moreover, "it's not certain whether
lactobacillus rhamnosus GG is effective in treating any
medical condition."(57)

▷ **In 2016,** science touted, "Psychobiotics will change the Hypothalamic-pituitary-adrenal axis."

▷ "The HPA circuit has long been recognized as an important regulatory loop between the brain and gut." (58)

The Hypothalamic-Pituitary-Adrenal Axis

A hypothalamic–pituitary–adrenal axis is said to be responsible for anxiety and depressive disorders. Chronic stress, and inflammation, disrupt the hypothalamus-pituitary-adrenal (HPA) axis, while imbalances in the hypothalamic-pituitary-adrenal axis are found common in mental illnesses. (59-60)

Consider the things that harm the hypothalamic-pituitary-adrenal axis are also endocrine disruptors, including environmental pollution, and heavy metals such as mercury. Mercury has disruptive effects on vitamin D absorption and on adrenal glands. (61) Mercury also crosses the blood brain-barrier, can accumulate in the central nervous system and contribute to oxidative stress. (62) Oxidative stress is then found in autoimmune disorders and depression.

"HPA axis activity is altered by obesity."(63) This means HPA activity is altered by poor food choices, poor sleep habits, and chronic stressful conditions, all contributing to obesity. (64-65)

Glucocorticoids

Scientists believe people exposed to chronic stress tend to have elevated levels of cortisol. (66) High cortisol levels can be dangerous to the brain, damages the lining of the gut, as well as raising blood sugar levels.

"Glucocorticoids, natural steroid (stress) hormones, do more than help the body respond to stress."(67) "They regulate physiological processes. (68) They also help the body respond to environmental change, glucose, and inflammation. In these roles, glucocorticoids are, in fact, essential for survival."

If we take a closer look at synthetic glucocorticoids, we see them used as anti-inflammatory drugs. (69) Research shows the administration of glucocorticoids to patients with normal adrenal function usually causes magnesium loss, irritability, insomnia, decreased cognition, and even psychosis. (70)

In adrenal fatigue, we may see mania and other disorders (such as anxiety) besides just psychotic symptoms. (71) However, we never have to wait for Big Pharma to step in. "More than 10 million new corticosteroid prescriptions are filled each year." (72) "Some are even absorbed in the nasal passage, which can directly target brain function." (73) Administration of Glucocorticoids can suppress the hypothalamic-pituitary-adrenal axis causing adrenal insufficiency in children. (74)

➡Cortisol affects emotional learning and memory processes. (75)

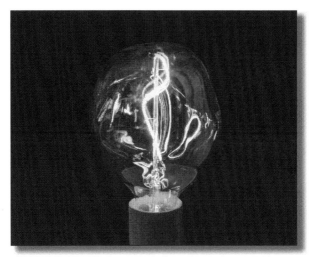

Epigenetic's Role in Gut/Brain Health

Epigenetic regulation can play a crucial role in the fate of the functioning of the immune system, good or bad. (76) Factors such as diet and exercise can be influential in immune system health and minimize disease. (77) If we understand which exposures can change our DNA and increase the risk for *Memory Stealers*, why do medical professionals stay silent?

In his book, *How Doctors Think*, physician and Harvard professor Jerome Groopman states, most doctors begin to make a diagnosis in the first few minutes of their assessment. Once this process begins, the doctor may dismiss symptoms that do not fit his preliminary diagnosis." If one is programmed to think, dismiss, or ignore the root cause of disease, one can cause irreparable harm.

In 2014 a growing body of evidence suggested that 'suicide vulnerability' may be due to epigenetic alterations in molecular pathways important for the hypothalamic-pituitary-adrenal (HPA) axis function."(78)

According to the Rowett Institute of Nutrition and Health and Karen P. Scott, "Our intestinal microbiota is an integral part of ourselves and cross-talk between the intestinal microbiota and the host." (79)

Finding clarity is found in the realization that toxic exposures we have been exposed to in the past and/or present can affect our descendants, and a SAD diet can change genes that are passed down through generations. (80)

The gist? The makings of mental illness (psychiatric disorders) and social anxiety disorders include epigenetic alterations. (81)

The Influence of DNA Methylation

• *DNA Methylation* Influences Gene Expression (83) Alcohol and smoking affect hepatic and neuronal tissue, disrupts neurotransmitters and causes *DNA methylation* changes. (84) The first step to changing an alcohol problem is to stop and ask for help.

• Heavy metals are capable of disrupting *DNA methylation* and, as a result, have been associated with a number of diseases, including neurological disorders and autoimmune diseases.

• "Sleep deprivation amongst adolescents is an epidemic. (85) Recent studies show that many adolescents maintain schedules during the school year that result in insufficient and ill-timed sleep." Sleep loss affects anxiety and depressive disorders and *DNA methylation* patterns. (86)

➡The good news is, when we make epigenetic modifications, there is great potential in inhibiting the progression of *Memory Stealers.* (82)

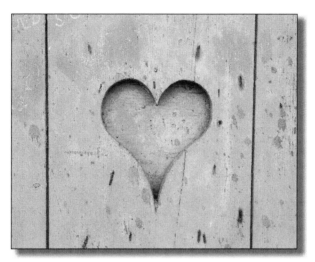

Who Stands To Win Using Psychobiotics?

Sigma-Aldrich: Makers of Dexamethasone, a cortisol medication with many side-effects. (87)

Eli Lilly & Co: Makers of Prozac with many side-effects. (88-89)

Syngenta on the board of directors for Eli Lilly. (90) Syngenta has been found to be part of Bayer/Monsanto Corporation. (91)

A Syngenta lawsuit settled in **2012** for 105 million for pollution of our waterways using Atrazine. (92) Studies found Atrazine is an endocrine disruptor, a substance that can alter the human hormonal system. It has the capacity to promote the epigenetic transgenerational inheritance of disease. (93)

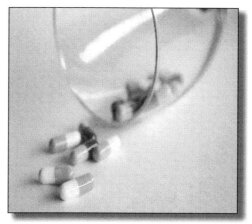

Antibiotics In Psychobiotics
Is it a Safety Concern?

▷ According to the Journal of Neuroscience, "Alterations from antibiotics are found in human brain diseases, including autism spectrum disorder, anxiety, depression, and chronic pain." (94)

▷ "Antibiotics stop the growth of brain cells."(95)

➤ According to Science Daily, "antibiotics strong enough to kill off gut bacteria can also harm brain cells in the hippocampus, a section of the brain associated with memory."[96] Changes in the hippocampus often accompany mental disorders. [97]

➤ "A short-term course of antibiotics may have a long-term negative impact on the human throat and gut microbiota."[98]

How Antibiotics Are Made

Antibiotics differ chemically depending on what bacterial disease they are designed to kill. From what I have studied, dangers can occur in the fermentation processes.

- ▷ One danger is, viruses can infect bacteria and fungi, passing along genes from one infected organism to the next. (99)

- ▷ They are made with ammonia salts. Ammonia Salt is where hydrochloric acid forms ammonium chloride. (100)

- ▷ They have a form of saprophytic bacteria, a fungus or bacterium, that lives and feeds on dead organic matter. (101)

- ▷ They may contain GMO soy meal and have several refining steps.

- ▷ They may contain dangerous microorganisms that are never listed on the label.

145

Memory Stealers

Plasma Homocysteine Levels & Mental Illness

In India, studies revealed, schizophrenia and depression are leading causes of morbidity in young adults. (102) It is well-known that mental stress elevates plasma homocysteine levels. (103)

Mental stress includes anxiety, depression, and neurological diseases, increasing high plasma levels of homocysteine. (104)

Additionally, alcohol addiction causes elevated plasma homocysteine levels, as does Metformin. (105) Metformin, a medication used to lower blood sugar, increases serum Hcy levels, and reduces B12 levels. (105a)

➡We can reduce our risk of Alzheimer's by reducing high homocysteine levels. Science tells us, the MTHFR gene is associated with elevated plasma homocysteine, which is detrimental to vascular integrity and has been linked to cognitive decline. (106a)

147

Assess Your Personal Risk

- Blood Pressure Imbalances

- Chronic Stress

- Lack of Sleep

- Obesity

- Smoking/Drinking

- Physical Inactivity

- Processed Foods

- A Toxic Environment

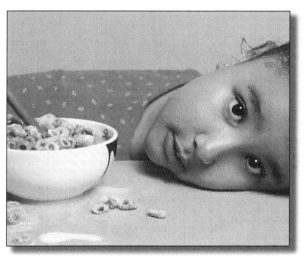

Trends

"With mental illness comes the power of convenience.
Convenience builds lazy. Lazy contributes to obesity, poor
cognition, and mental disorders." CR

Trends That Lower Cognition

▷ Five to six hours a day spent watching television. A
sedentary lifestyle increases our risk for cognitive
impairment, stress, and overeating.

▶ Junk food restaurants are fast, convent, easy, and have toxic scents throughout. They leave us craving for more processed foods, increasing our risk for poor gut microbiome and mental instability.

▶ Bottled water, colored water, vitamin water, and drinks in plastic containers contribute to toxic waterways, toxic foods, and air pollution. This plastic lifestyle increases our risk for behavioral issues and poor mental health.

▶ New and convenient household cleaners containing what I call 'death scents' are causal in central nervous system disorders, brain disorders, skin disorders, and other organ toxicities. These do not clean the air we breathe; they pollute it instead. I visited a neighbors house where she had two large dogs, and as I walked in, I discovered six plug-ins air-fresheners in her home. (one in each room) She washed her floors with Pine-Sol. After a few minutes, I couldn't breathe and had to remove myself from her home.

▷ Bariatric surgery, an easy way to lose unwanted weight. Studies suggest bariatric surgery may compromise your mental health."(106)

▷ We are fed misinformation on why boxed dead foods are a great food for breakfast. The lies include fiber-rich, enriched, low-fat, whole grain, and good for your heart! In reality, they are all loaded with processed sugars that are not good for the heart. And now, quick and easy breakfast cereals can even contain glyphosate.

➡Exposure to glyphosate changes gut microbiome and is found causal in mental disorders and premature births. (107-108)

Memory Stealers

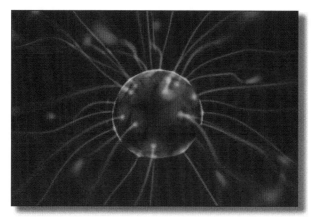

Impaired Neurotransmitters & Mental Illness

"Researchers seem to agree that key players responsible for the bacteria-gut-brain axis are the nervous system of the intestines, the immune system, the vagus nerve, gut hormones, and neurotransmitters."

What Harms Key Players?

▷ "According to Dr. Richard Wurtman at MIT, who is involved in numerous studies on nutrition and the brain, "the nutrients in foods are precursors to neurotransmitters, and depending on the number of precursors present in the food you eat, the more or less of a certain neurotransmitter is produced." "Neurotransmitters carry signals to your brain and body. When impaired, depression and other emotional disorders occur."

▷ Antidepressants can alter neurotransmitters.

▷ "Scientists have found that gut bacteria produce neurotransmitters such as serotonin, dopamine, and GABA, and play a key role in mood and mental health." (109) When we consume benzodiazepines (Benzos), these affect GABA in the brain by reducing activity.

▷ In my previous chapters, you'll see *stress* can cause sleep deprivation. In the United States alone, approximately

154

25% of children do not get sufficient sleep, making them prone to adult diseases. (112-113)

▶ Stress also alters GABA. "GABA is an inhibitory neurotransmitter in the central nervous system." (110) Prolonged stress and cortisol imbalances lead us to obesity, *Memory Stealers*, mental instability, and diabetes. (111)

▶ Corporations believe, we need to fix cortisol imbalances with better medications. In the U.S., Corcept Therapeutics Inc, a pharmaceutical company, is responsible for the development of cortisol modulators. (114-115)

▶ "When neurotransmitters are disrupted by pollution, the reaction creates an increased risk for oxidative stress and central nervous system disorders, insomnia, and mental illness, including delirium." (116-118)

▷ Dopamine changes when exposed to pesticides. "Dopamine is a neurotransmitter that activates pleasure centers in certain areas of the brain." Our brain makes and uses dopamine. Atrazine, a pesticide, is sprayed on soy and corn crops and golf courses and is found in our waterways. Atrazine adversely affects the brain dopaminergic system and is found to be extremely toxic to our brain cells. This toxicity increases the risk of mental instability. (119-120)

▷ Oral contraceptive use can decrease serotonin levels and increase cortisol levels. Other studies show, 'oral contraceptives increase the risk for mental illness in young women." (121)

▷ Contrave, a prescription weight loss/diet pill, contains an opioid antagonist and an antidepressant. Side-effects may include neuropsychiatric behavior, constipation, headache, anxiety, UTI, HBP, and changes in tastes. (114a)

Here, I'll discuss only two foods that impair neurotransmitter production. (there are many more) Opioid peptides from dairy and wheat-related products. In dairy products, we can find growth hormones and the protein casein. In wheat, we may find Cycocel, a synthetic hormone growth regulator, and pesticides such as malathion.

➡Levels of neurotransmitters in the brain and gut are easily manipulated. Children need fewer toxins, not more drugs, in order to create balance.

Memory Stealers

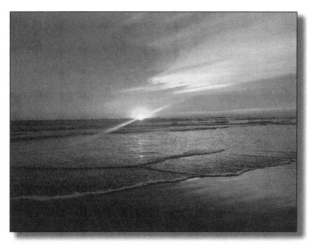

The Long Search for Balance

What we know to be true helps determine balance.

▷ Research shows we can rebuild our brains with the foods we put in our gut. (122) We can change its function and structure throughout our entire life.

▷ Children need to get more sleep, not less. Metabolic syndrome, obesity, and type 2 diabetes have a direct relationship with insomnia, dementia, poor gut microbes, and poor mental health. Insomnia can increase stress, and stress can increase insomnia. "About 50 to 70 million Americans suffer from sleep disorders."[123]

▶ The gut microbiome is responsible for healthy neurotransmitters. Deficiencies in neurotransmitters negatively impact moods. Health is a choice!

▶ Making brain-drain a thing of the past is something to consider *every* day of your life. Our brain is the most important organ in our body, and we need to treat it as such. Our gut and brain work in tandem, each influencing the other. We taste and enjoy life *WHEN* these two organs communicate well!

There is a significant breakthrough, on why we need to feed the mind with excellent self-care habits. It's *BECAUSE* all habits will affect our very survival.

It seems crazy that social shyness, social phobias, mood changes, and anxiety can be all lumped together to form new pharmaceuticals. "The pharmaceutical industry has corrupted the practice of medicine through its influence over what drugs are developed, how they are tested, marketed, and how medical knowledge is created." (124) Make no mistake; Big Pharma spends millions each year lobbying politicians. We have a society that invests billions in creating *unconsciousness* to ensure we stay lost.

➡Wouldn't it be healthier to eat foods first? The answer is, Yes.

Nothing could be more serious than the disrupted nature of poor nutrition, poor gut microbiome, and the things that poison and kill brain cells. (125) The end results are increased fears, phobias, and chances of losing our mind.

.

.

Chapter 4

The Mind & Kidney Connection

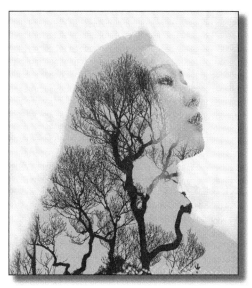

An Opportunity To Heal

"Chronic low-grade inflammation is a hallmark of Chronic Kidney Disease, and has been disclosed as one important factor contributing to the progression of CKD and high cardiovascular mortality."

According to Executive Order by President Trump on July 10th 2019, "Within 120 days of the date of this order, the Secretary of Health and Human Services shall launch an awareness initiative at the Department of Health and Human Services to aid the Secretary's efforts to educate patients and support programs that promote kidney disease awareness. The initiative shall develop proposals for the Secretary to support research regarding preventing, treating, and slowing the progression of kidney disease; to improve kidney transplantation, and to share information with patients and providers to enhance awareness of the causes and consequences of kidney disease."

"Kidney disease was the ninth leading cause of death in the United States in 2017. Approximately 37 million Americans have Chronic Kidney Disease, and more than 726,000 have End-Stage Renal Disease."

So, the question is, how do we promote awareness and prevent kidney disease or renal failure?

I've investigated and researched many contributors to this deadly disease. What I've discovered is, Chronic Kidney Disease (CKD) is a byproduct of toxic exposures involved in *Memory Stealers*. Yes, it's true! This means what we eat, drink, medicate, and surround ourselves with, supersedes genetics.

To enjoy excellent health, it's all about balance. With just a few lifestyle changes, we can prevent and reverse kidney disease (1) and achieve homeostasis.

Memory Stealers

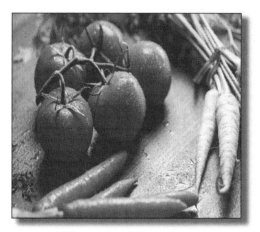

Changing The Course

Chronic Kidney Disease is identified more commonly among patients with severe mental illness than in the general population and is associated with a higher cardiovascular risk. (55)

About 50% of Veterans suffer from Chronic Kidney Disease. One of the requirements for men going to war is to receive vaccinations. Studies acknowledge that Veterans in the Gulf war were given multiple dirty vaccines containing toxic chemicals and heavy metals. (27) They we not allowed to question what was in them.

In reality, mercury, and other heavy metals accumulate readily in the kidneys. (28)

"The CDC reports that as many as 80 million Americans are insulin resistant, and most do not pay attention to insulin resistance being a precursor to diabetes."(4) Not only is insulin resistance associated with HBP and PCOS, (39) it can also adversely affect all organs in the body, including the kidneys! When connecting the dots, I found insulin resistance and cardiovascular disease promotes the rapid progression of Chronic Kidney Disease. (5) Why? Because our heart works in tandem with our kidneys, what affects one affects the other. Other influencers increasing our risk factors for kidney disease are smoking, obesity, *Memory Stealers*, and hypertension. (2-3)

- The good news is "weight loss and reduction of belly fat almost invariably reverses insulin resistance."(6)

Hypertension is one cause of Chronic Kidney Disease. "Cortisol is a vital catabolic hormone produced by the adrenal cortex of the kidney."(9) Cortisol helps regular metabolism and blood sugar levels. Cortisol imbalances can be found causal in low energy levels, constipation, insomnia, depression, and often indicate adrenal fatigue. (10-11) The adrenal glands sit on top of our kidneys and are a part of our endocrine system. What disrupts our endocrine system disrupts our kidney health.

Balancing cortisol levels can protect the body from adrenal fatigue. (12)

Memory Stealers

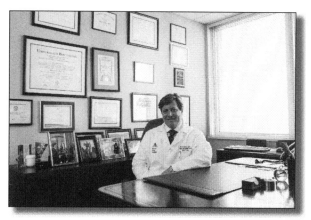

Medications Linked to Kidney Disease

- Metformin is marketed as a diabetic medication with side-effects, including lactic acidosis, decreased vitamin B12 levels, coma, and difficulty in urination.

- HRT has an association with poor kidney health. (13)

- Statins have an association with acute kidney injury. (14) Chronic use of statins induces insulin resistance and diabetes plus have side-effects that include heart disease, aggression, and weight gain. (15) Some studies even suggest there is a lack of evidence that statins even prevent heart disease. (16)

- Zoloft may decrease kidney function, making kidney disease [17] worse. Additionally, SSRI's/interrupt metabolism, gut microbiome and can increase the risk of obesity.

- Opioids [18] claim over 400,000 lives a year. "Toxic substances such as opioids prevent the body from the natural filtering and elimination processes. When kidneys become damaged, hormone levels are also imbalanced, and we can no longer excrete waste properly."

- Anti-inflammatories such as sulfasalazine (Azulfidine) have side-effects, including kidney stones.

- Humira [19] is an injectable protein used to treat arthritis, psoriasis, and Crohn's disease. Side-effects include kidney calculus (kidney stones).

- Abilify is used to treat schizophrenia and bipolar disorders. Side-effects include kidney disease. [20]

- Avastin is taken for age-related macular degeneration, and side-effects include vision loss and retinal detachment. "This happens because of this drug, possibly causing too much protein in the urine."[21]

- "Researchers want better warning labels, for Rolaids, Tums, Prilosec, and other producers of antacids."(21a-b) Some side-effects for Prilosec include bone fractures to kidney dangers.

Noteworthy: Obese and depressed individuals may juggle more than five medications a day. It's time to ask questions surrounding the interactions between specific medications, depression, and obesity and how they increase our risk for kidney disease.

Memory Stealers

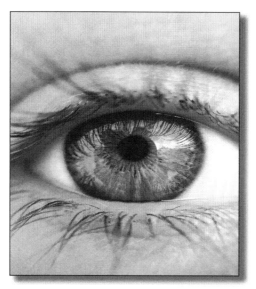

The Kidney Eye Connection

Our eyes are a window to our kidneys. (22) In Chinese medicine, (23) there are meridians from the eyes to the kidneys. "When the meridians are flowing smoothly, there is neither pain nor illness. When blockages exist in meridians, pain, and illness result." Increased Age-Related Macular Degeneration is common among individuals with reduced kidney function. (24)

Macular degeneration comorbidities can be associated with heart disease and diabetes. (25)

➡ Acupuncture treatments, avoiding sugary foods, and making sure you are never dehydrated can help symptoms of macular degeneration.

The Kidney Gut Connection

It's no surprise that kidney disease is directly linked to diabetes, with diabetes, eventually leading to kidney cancer. It may be interesting to find the cause is related to diet. Daily consumption of sugar feeds diabetes, Alzheimer's, CVD, and Chronic Kidney Disease. (7-8) Moreover, if that doesn't grab your attention, High Fructose Corn Syrup changes brain cells, increases cravings, and increases our risk factor for the beginnings of renal inflammation! (see pg 79)

Wireless Radiation and EMF exposures may fuel estrogen dominance.

There's an interconnection between estrogen dominance and obesity, linking it to kidney cancer. (35-36) Estrogen dominance is linked to the bombardment of xenoestrogens which impair immunity, and create hormonal imbalances. Xenoestrogens have disruptive effects in oral health and gut health. Both Chronic Kidney Disease and estrogen dominance are associated with multiple physiological and metabolic disturbances. (37) This is because the gut microbiome is the ecosystem of bacteria that lives inside us that not only influences the development of estrogen dominance but also participates in the etiology of CVD. (38)

"The interaction between gut microbiota and Chronic Kidney Disease is not unidirectional. Chronic Kidney Disease affects the structure of the gut microbiota and visa versa."(43) Deficiency in gut microbes and the increase in free radical damage leads us down the road to preventable health issues, including kidney disorders!

Some foods that are toxic to our organs and our endocrine system don't require a warning label. Take for instance vegetable oils. Vegetable oils are linked to most inflammatory conditions including metabolic syndrome. Choosing healthier oils, such as organic olive oil, is also better for cognitive function.

Globally unaddressed is the frequent use of energy drinks/ caffeinated drinks and other nervous system stimulants that create imbalances in adrenals and irritate renal function. Energy drinks keep the body in a dehydrated state. In 2020 Coke™ has provided us with a new, improved energy drink. In a 16oz serving, it may contain a whopping 152 mg of caffeine. Some other ingredients listed include dextrose and natural flavorings.

• Making simple dietary changes, working through stress, and avoiding stimulants, such as energy drinks, can be three steps toward changing the course of Chronic Kidney Disease.

Pesticides & Kidney Function

We are a nation suffering from an abundance of pesticides and heavy metal exposures known to be carcinogenic. Pesticides and chemicals are found to be risk factors for kidney cancer. (29-30) To make this risk factor recognizable, we can make a note as to how many of our friends set off roach bombs in their kitchen every six months.

Pesticides are a considerable risk factor for Veterans that fought in Vietnam, The Gulf War, and the Iraq War. (26)

Long term side-effects from DDT, Agent Orange, and others include, but are not limited to, kidney disease, eye disease, and cardiovascular disease.

According to Autoimmunity Research Foundation from 2012, "The rate of chronic disease in the U.S. has been dramatically increasing over the years from environmental triggers rather than genetic or age-related causes."(49)

- Glyphosate is an environmental trigger. It drives the obesity epidemic and the cancer epidemic. It's also causal in brain fog. The Journal of Public Health And Emergency states there is even an association between heart disease and glyphosate. (50) And, today we know Monsanto's glyphosate spent the last 30+ years covering up kidney cancers. Environmental Pollution is significantly associated with increased risk of type 2 diabetes and other major preventable diseases. (52) Moreover, according to the Lancet, Pollution is the most significant environmental cause of illnesses to all organs. (53)

• According to Journal of Organic Systems, glyphosate plays a role in kidney cancer and acute kidney failure. (51) Once again, environmental pollution is the most significant cause of disease. "Glyphosate can cause a cascade of metabolic and homeostatic changes that result in catastrophic renal damage."(48)

"According to BeyondPesticides.org, glyphosate substitution for glycine correlates with several diseases, including kidney disease, diabetes, obesity, Alzheimer's disease, and Parkinson's disease, among others." (53a)

➡The good news is that we are finally beginning to see the light at the end of the tunnel, however small of a difference we make. More than 13,000 have file lawsuits against Monsanto. Changing exposures to environmental pollution can influence changing the course of kidney disease.

Memory Stealers

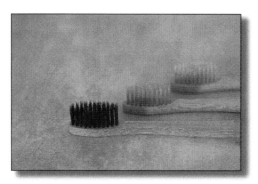

Kidneys & Oral Health

Periodontal disease is a seriously overlooked problem putting a strain on our kidneys. (31) In holistic dentistry, which is becoming more popular, teeth have a synergistic and meridian connection to vital organs. (32) Chronic kidney disease also has a strong association with periodontal disease. (33) Poor kidney health is just one consequence when we do not pay attention to proper oral health.

- Poor oral health and kidney disease can and will negatively affect diabetes, Alzheimer's, and CVD. (34)

Noteworthy: There is a positive association between fluoride and kidney disease. (44) Fluoride can be found in processed foods, wine, tap water, bottled water, toothpaste, and the list goes on. Fluoride has also been linked to thyroid problems. (45) The Catch? Thyroid dysfunction affects renal physiology and development, and kidney disease could result in thyroid dysfunction. (46)

Christopher Bryson's widely acclaimed book *"The Fluoride Deception,"* includes dozens of peer-reviewed studies showing that sodium fluoride is a deadly neurotoxin that attacks the central nervous system and leads to a multitude of severe health problems. (see more on Fluoride Page 97)

Kidneys & Sun Exposure

Natural sun exposure, but not a sunburn, is critical for all life on this planet. As humans, we can not live without sunshine! Studies have demonstrated a link between vitamin D deficiency and Chronic Kidney Disease mortality in the general population. (46a-b) "Too much vitamin D, or Hypervitaminosis D, can result from a high-dosed vitamin D supplementation used for several months. Overdoing Vitamin D supplements can lead to high blood pressure, bone loss, and kidney damage."(47)

Memory Stealers

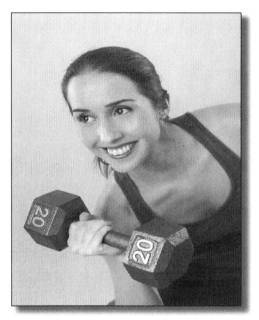

Slow The Progression of Kidney Disease

If we want to slow the progression of kidney disease, we must first take a serious look at the multiple causes!

As you can see by know, Metabolic Syndrome is a risk factor that accelerates the progression of kidney disease. If we slow the progression of CVD, Diabetes, HBP, Insulin Resistance, and others, we can change the way we treat renal disease. We can do this by understanding and uncovering the hidden connections between foods, medications, environmental triggers, and how big our body burden is when attempting to eliminate toxins. (53)

We can gather together and find ways to become active in changing laws that no longer protect us within the EPA and FDA. We can also find a way to keep our body and brain active. Exercise is a significant influencer in changing the course of kidney disease.

Over the last 15+ years, Chronic Kidney Disease has increased in children. Sadly, there is a correlation between growth impairment and mineral and bone disorders in children with Chronic Kidney Disease. (54)

Hopefully, this gets your attention. It got mine!

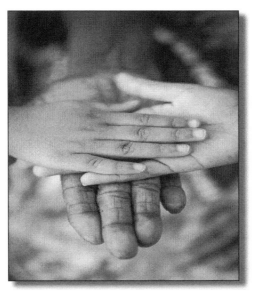

Connie's Immune Recovery Program
10 years from now, will You lose YOU?

Researchers at the University of Virginia School of Medicine have determined that our brain is directly connected to our immune system! This 2015 discovery has changed the way people look at the central nervous system's relationship and communication with the immune system. To clarify, this means neuroinflammatory and neurodegenerative diseases are associated with immune system dysfunction.

189

What occurs in our immune system occurs in our brain!

*There's compelling evidence for the existence of fungal proteins in brain samples from Alzheimer's disease patients.

*A stressed immune system can create negative changes in hormones and weight balance.

*Declining lung health can be considered a predictor of cognitive decline.

*A stellar immune system doesn't have room for toxic moods. Weak immunity, poor behavior, agitation, depression, and brain atrophy are found in people with Alzheimer's.

Self-neglect and toxic exposures can steal our memories, our taste buds, our friends, our family, our heart, our collagen and elastin, our energy reserves and depress our immune system before we are 50 years old.

It's time to make a difference rather than a disability!

I invite you to join my '*Immune System Recovery Program*'-because finding new ways to make your mental health a priority, is priceless! Thank you.

For more information, go to:

https://bitesizepieces.lpages.co/steps-to-get-toxins-out/

Take Action to improve your brain power. Set up a consultation to speak with me today. faces@vail.net

Connie Rogers is a Published Author, Writer, Professional Researcher, Health Coach & Brain Health Coach. She is an expert in teaching holistic options to empower you to take action steps for gut & brain health. Author of *MEMORY STEALERS & Other Illusions!*

DISCLAIMER.....

The content of this book is for general instruction only. Each person's physical, emotional, and spiritual condition is unique. The instruction in this book is not intended to replace or interrupt the reader's relationship with a physician or other professional. Please consult your doctor for matters pertaining to your specific health and dietary needs.

Memory Stealers

Memory Stealers & Other Illusions
Footnotes

1-https://www.ncbi.nlm.nih.gov/pmc/articles/PMC5266861/

2- https://www.ncbi.nlm.nih.gov/pmc/articles/PMC4228144/

3- www.ncbi.nlm.nih.gov/pubmed/16340083

4-https://www.ncbi.nlm.nih.gov/pmc/articles/PMC5834839/

5-https://www.ncbi.nlm.nih.gov/pubmed/27651175

5a-https://www.npr.org/sections/health-shots/2017/07/16/536935957/stress-and-poverty-may-explain-high-rates-of-dementia-in-african-americans

6- https://www.ncbi.nlm.nih.gov/pmc/articles/PMC4847540/

7- http://www.movement-of-life.org/2016/06/16/this-drug-in-your-medicine-cabinet-shrinks-brains/

8-http://www.naturalnews.com/053835_OTC_medication_cognitive_impairment_anticholinergic_drugs.html#ixzz47ypD7XbO

9-https://www.ncbi.nlm.nih.gov/pubmed/18483351

10-http://medicalxpress.com/news/2014-06-loss-brain-vulnerability-toxic-elements.html

11-https://www.ncbi.nlm.nih.gov/pubmed/18363822

12- https://www.health.harvard.edu/mind-and-mood/two-types-of-drugs-you-may-want-to-avoid-for-the-sake-of-your-brain see also https://www.sciencedaily.com/releases/2018/04/180425195636.htm

13-https://www.pharmacytimes.com/publications/issue/2008/2008-11/2008-11-8747

14-http://drkaayladaniel.com/the-poop-on-miralax/

15-www.rxlist.com/nausea/symptoms.htm

16-www.rxlist.com/dizziness_dizzy/article.htm

17-https://pdfs.semanticscholar.org/e57c/b8de87a7ebe5613cebd261339e2fc3fdff39.pdf

18-https://www.ncbi.nlm.nih.gov/pmc/articles/PMC2836429/

19-http://www.ncbi.nlm.nih.gov/pubmed/9470898

19a-https://www.mdedge.com/psychiatry/article/77689/anxiety-disorders/problematic-pruritus-seeking-cure-psychogenic-itch

19b-https://www.ncbi.nlm.nih.gov/pmc/articles/PMC4270264/

20-https://www.ncbi.nlm.nih.gov/pubmed/28614811

21-https://www.ncbi.nlm.nih.gov/pmc/articles/PMC3018626/

22-https://www.ncbi.nlm.nih.gov/pmc/articles/PMC4273443/

23-https://www.ncbi.nlm.nih.gov/pubmed/6123986

24-https://www.ncbi.nlm.nih.gov/books/NBK47449/ see also https://www.ncbi.nlm.nih.gov/pubmed/12115887 the enemy within https://www.ncbi.nlm.nih.gov/pubmed/18487848

25- https://www.ncbi.nlm.nih.gov/pmc/articles/PMC4221694/

26- www.ncbi.nlm.nih.gov/pubmed/24313931

27-https://www.ncbi.nlm.nih.gov/pubmed/27589534

28-https://www.ncbi.nlm.nih.gov/pubmed/29676229

29-https://www.ncbi.nlm.nih.gov/pmc/articles/PMC6066504/

30-https://www.ncbi.nlm.nih.gov/pubmed/24614898

31-https://www.ncbi.nlm.nih.gov/pmc/articles/PMC2831066/?

32-https://www.ncbi.nlm.nih.gov/pmc/articles/PMC6288487/

33-https://www.ncbi.nlm.nih.gov/pmc/articles/PMC5652018/

34-https://www.ncbi.nlm.nih.gov/pubmed/25230225

35-https://www.ncbi.nlm.nih.gov/pmc/articles/PMC3171359/?

36-https://www.ncbi.nlm.nih.gov/pmc/articles/PMC6288487/

36a-https://www.mc.vanderbilt.edu/reporter/index.html?ID=779

37-https://www.ncbi.nlm.nih.gov/pmc/articles/PMC6022993/

38-https://www.ncbi.nlm.nih.gov/pubmed/15059276

39-https://www.ncbi.nlm.nih.gov/pubmed/27111329

40-https://www.ncbi.nlm.nih.gov/pubmed/27111329

41-https://academic.oup.com/jid/article-pdf/
174/2/424/2492118/174-2-424.pdf

42-https://www.ncbi.nlm.nih.gov/pubmed/25922779/

43-https://www.ommegaonline.org/article-details/Lyme-disease-and-
dementia-Alzheimer-Parkinson-Autism-an-easy-way-to-destroy-your-
brain/1992

44-https://www.ncbi.nlm.nih.gov/pubmed/7943444

45-https://jamanetwork.com/journals/jama/article-abstract/362744

46-https://ecfsapi.fcc.gov/file/7520958029.pdf

47-https://subtle.energy/the-schumann-effect-how-the-earth-influences-your-brain/

48-https://www.ncbi.nlm.nih.gov/pubmed/29718124

49-https://www.ncbi.nlm.nih.gov/pubmed/30481957

50-https://n.neurology.org/content/47/6/1594

51-https://ecfsapi.fcc.gov/file/7520958029.pdf

52-https://www.ncbi.nlm.nih.gov/pubmed/12843764

53-https://news.usc.edu/12202/Study-Finds-Electromagnetic-Fields-May-Increase-Risk-of-Alzheimer-s/

54-http://www.ncbi.nlm.nih.gov/pmc/articles/PMC4380045/

55-http://www.ncbi.nlm.nih.gov/pubmed/23051584/

56-https://www.ncbi.nlm.nih.gov/pubmed/24053962

56a-https://www.ncbi.nlm.nih.gov/pubmed/8012056?dopt=Abstract

57-https://www.sciencedirect.com/science/article/pii/S0891061815000599

58-https://www.ncbi.nlm.nih.gov/pmc/articles/PMC3323189/

59-https://www.ncbi.nlm.nih.gov/pmc/articles/PMC4010966/

59a-https://www.ncbi.nlm.nih.gov/pmc/articles/PMC3216414/

60-https://www.ncbi.nlm.nih.gov/pmc/articles/PMC5551541/

61-https://www.ncbi.nlm.nih.gov/pmc/articles/PMC2724665/

62-https://www.ncbi.nlm.nih.gov/pmc/articles/PMC4938117/

63-https://www.ncbi.nlm.nih.gov/pubmed/22884479

64-https://www.ncbi.nlm.nih.gov/pubmed/21971457

65-https://www.fda.gov/ForConsumers/ConsumerUpdates/ucm048919.htm

66-www.medicalnewstoday.com/articles/294616.php

67-https://www.ncbi.nlm.nih.gov/pmc/articles/PMC6282746/

68-articles.mercola.com/sites/articles/archive/2010/04/24/epstein-interview.aspx

69-https://www.ncbi.nlm.nih.gov/pubmed/20545755

70-https://www.ncbi.nlm.nih.gov/pmc/articles/PMC5400116/

71-https://www.ncbi.nlm.nih.gov/pmc/articles/PMC3967436/

72-https://www.ncbi.nlm.nih.gov/pmc/articles/PMC2957945/

73-https://cspinet.org/sites/default/files/attachment/food-dyes-rainbow-of-risks.pdf

73a-https://www.ncbi.nlm.nih.gov/pubmed/20667460

74a-https://www.ncbi.nlm.nih.gov/pubmed/1579515

74-http://www.ncbi.nlm.nih.gov/pubmed/11684540

75-https://www.ncbi.nlm.nih.gov/pmc/articles/PMC6198681/

76-https://www.ncbi.nlm.nih.gov/pmc/articles/PMC3262151/

77-http://www.bmj.com/content/349/bmj.g5205

78-https://link.springer.com/article/10.1007/s12325-012-0050-8

78a- https://www.biography.com/news/robin-williams-mind-life-death

78b-https://n.neurology.org/content/64/5/861

78c-https://molecularneurodegeneration.biomedcentral.com/articles/
10.1186/s13024-019-0306-8

79-https://www.who.int/news-room/detail/13-09-2019-who-calls-for-
urgent-action-to-reduce-patient-harm-in-healthcare

79a- https://www.ncbi.nlm.nih.gov/m/pubmed/25882659/?
i=3&from=pemf therapy circulation

80-https://www.ncbi.nlm.nih.gov/pubmed/25196099?dopt=Abstract

80a- https://www.ncbi.nlm.nih.gov/pubmed/25271249

81-https://www.ncbi.nlm.nih.gov/books/NBK507908/

82-https://www.ncbi.nlm.nih.gov/pubmed/21126996

83-https://www.ncbi.nlm.nih.gov/pmc/articles/PMC5594560/

84-https://www.ncbi.nlm.nih.gov/pmc/articles/PMC4266989/

85-http://gut.bmj.com/content/43/4/506.full

85a-https://www.ncbi.nlm.nih.gov/pubmed/29169241

86-https://www.ncbi.nlm.nih.gov/pmc/articles/PMC6313445/

86a- https://www.uptodate.com/contents/nsaids-including-aspirin-
pathogenesis-of-gastroduodenal-toxicity

87-https://www.ncbi.nlm.nih.gov/pubmed/29892317

87a- https://www.ncbi.nlm.nih.gov/pubmed/9667488

87b- http://npic.orst.edu/ingred/ptype/mothball/health.html

88-https://www.mentalhelp.net/blogs/benzodiazepine-use-linked-to-
alzheimer-s-disease/

89-https://www.frontiersin.org/articles/10.3389/fnint.2013.00086/full

90-https://www.ncbi.nlm.nih.gov/pmc/articles/PMC4082169/

91-https://www.ncbi.nlm.nih.gov/pmc/articles/PMC3051846/

92-https://www.ncbi.nlm.nih.gov/pmc/articles/PMC4062078/

93-https://www.gastrojournal.org/article/S0016-5085(16)34319-0/fulltext

94-https://www.ncbi.nlm.nih.gov/pmc/articles/PMC4423197/

95-https://www.ncbi.nlm.nih.gov/pmc/articles/PMC4126236/

96-https://www.ncbi.nlm.nih.gov/pmc/articles/PMC3669067/

97-https://www.ncbi.nlm.nih.gov/pubmed/27397854

98-https://www.ncbi.nlm.nih.gov/pmc/articles/PMC3548567/

99-https://www.ncbi.nlm.nih.gov/pmc/articles/PMC6127743/

100- https://www.ncbi.nlm.nih.gov/pmc/articles/PMC3951193/

101-https://www.ncbi.nlm.nih.gov/pmc/articles/PMC3951193/

102-https://www.ncbi.nlm.nih.gov/pmc/articles/PMC1993986/

102a-https://www.niehs.nih.gov/health/topics/agents/endocrine/index.cfm

103-http://nonhazcity.eu/wp-content/uploads/2018/11/brochure_plastics_EN_web-ilovepdf-compressed.pdf

104-https://www.ncbi.nlm.nih.gov/pmc/articles/PMC5328683/

104a- https://www.ncbi.nlm.nih.gov/pmc/articles/PMC4112067/

105-https://www.ncbi.nlm.nih.gov/pmc/articles/PMC3317180/

106-journals.plos.org/plosone/article?id=10.1371/journal.pone.0145274

106a-https://www.ncbi.nlm.nih.gov/pmc/articles/PMC1476028/

106b-https://www.ncbi.nlm.nih.gov/pubmed/12086542

107-https://www.ncbi.nlm.nih.gov/pubmed/30173377

107a-https://onlinelibrary.wiley.com/doi/abs/10.1002/eat.22397

108-https://www.ncbi.nlm.nih.gov/pubmed/25402818

109-https://www.ncbi.nlm.nih.gov/pmc/articles/PMC4468824/

110-https://www.sciencedaily.com/releases/2012/04/120402162546.htm

110a-https://www.ncoa.org/wp-content/uploads/
Depression_Older_Persons_FactSheet_2009.pdf

111- https://www.biorxiv.org/content/10.1101/673350v3.full

112-https://www.ncbi.nlm.nih.gov/pmc/articles/PMC4434967/

112a- https://www.who.int/features/qa/27/en/

112a- https://windheimemfsolutions.com/wp-content/uploads/2014/08/
EHS-Presentation-Steve-Weller.pdf

113- http://www.ncbi.nlm.nih.gov/pmc/articles/PMC1940091/

114-https://www.ncbi.nlm.nih.gov/pubmed/18473848

115-https://www.ncbi.nlm.nih.gov/pmc/articles/PMC5266861/

116-https://www.researchgate.net/publication/
330514782_Food_advanced_glycation_end_products_as_potential_endo
crine_disruptors_An_emerging_threat_to_contemporary_and_future_ge
neration

117-https://www.mdpi.com/2218-273X/9/12/888/htm

118-https://link.springer.com/chapter/10.1007/978-4-431-54490-6_3

118a-https://www.ncbi.nlm.nih.gov/pubmed/16594265

119-https://www.ncbi.nlm.nih.gov/pmc/articles/PMC2738337/

120-https://www.ncbi.nlm.nih.gov/pmc/articles/PMC6313445/

121-www.ei-resource.org/illness-information/environmental-illnesses/leaky-gut-syndrome-(lgs)/

122-https://www.ncbi.nlm.nih.gov/pmc/articles/PMC6052050/

123-https://www.ncbi.nlm.nih.gov/pmc/articles/PMC5793908/

124-www.diseaseproof.com/archives/healthy-pregnancy-coumadin-vitamin-k-and-a-plantbased-diet.html

125- https://www.jneurosci.org/content/36/28/7428

126- https://www.ncbi.nlm.nih.gov/pmc/articles/PMC5213281/

127-https://link.springer.com/article/10.1007/s00540-019-02623-7

128-http://www.ncbi.nlm.nih.gov/pubmed/19580862

129- https://www.ncbi.nlm.nih.gov/pubmed/21504113

139-https://www.ncbi.nlm.nih.gov/pubmed/30348620?

131-https://www.ncbi.nlm.nih.gov/pubmed/24769037

132-https://journals.physiology.org/doi/full/10.1152/jn.01075.2009

133-https://www.ncbi.nlm.nih.gov/pubmed/29346115

133a- https://www.sciencedaily.com/releases/2017/12/171206132526.htm

134-https://www.ncbi.nlm.nih.gov/pmc/articles/PMC3317180/

135-https://www.ncbi.nlm.nih.gov/pubmed/15563910

136-https://www.ncbi.nlm.nih.gov/pubmed/18349428/

136a- https://www.the-scientist.com/features/what-sensory-receptors-do-outside-of-sense-organs-32942

137-https://www.ncbi.nlm.nih.gov/pubmed/12619779/

138-https://www.ncbi.nlm.nih.gov/pmc/articles/PMC3471510/

138a https://www.ncbi.nlm.nih.gov/pubmed/21280072

139-https://www.researchgate.net/publication/294726215_Effect_of_Long_Term_Administration_of_Aspartame_on_the_Ultrastructure_of_Sciatic_Nerve_of_Adult_Male_Albino_Rat

140-https://www.ncbi.nlm.nih.gov/pmc/articles/PMC4199287/

141-https://neuropathycommons.org/neuropathy/neuropathy-sleep

142-https://www.spandidos-publications.com/10.3892/ijmm.2019.4142

143-https://www.ncbi.nlm.nih.gov/pmc/articles/PMC4528905/

144-https://www.ncbi.nlm.nih.gov/pmc/articles/PMC5942574/

145-http://www.ncbi.nlm.nih.gov/pmc/articles/PMC2856357/

146-https://www.ncbi.nlm.nih.gov/pubmed/30225985

147-https://www.jneurosci.org/content/28/14/3689

148-https://www.ncbi.nlm.nih.gov/pmc/articles/PMC2585730/

149-www.scielo.br/scielo.php?script=sci_arttext&pid=S1516-89132010000600008

150-https://www.ncbi.nlm.nih.gov/pubmed/30312575

151-https://www.ncbi.nlm.nih.gov/pmc/articles/PMC4310835/

152-www.visionaware.org/info/your-eye-condition/age-related-macular-degeneration-amd/risk-factors-for-amd/125

153-https://www.omicsonline.org/neuroinflammation-and-neurodegenerative-disorders-of-the-retina-2161-1017.1000111.php?

154-https://www.ncbi.nlm.nih.gov/pubmed/28402535

155-https://www.ncbi.nlm.nih.gov/pmc/articles/PMC4152129/

156-www.ncbi.nlm.nih.gov/pubmed/12796248

157-https://www.brightfocus.org/common-features-neurodegenerative-diseases-exploring-brain-eye-connection-and-beyond-1

158-www.nutritionalmagnesium.org/does-magnesium-supplementation-improve-muscle-health/

159-https://www.ncbi.nlm.nih.gov/pmc/articles/PMC5551541/

160-https://www.sciencedirect.com/science/article/pii/S1350946217301271

161-https://www.ncbi.nlm.nih.gov/pmc/articles/PMC3880532/

162-https://www.ncbi.nlm.nih.gov/pubmed/15730230

163-https://www.ncbi.nlm.nih.gov/pmc/articles/PMC3708350/

164-https://www.sciencedirect.com/book/9780124017177/handbook-of-nutrition-diet-and-the-eye

165-https://www.niams.nih.gov/newsroom/spotlight-on-research/bone-hormone-found-influence-brain-development

166-https://www.ncbi.nlm.nih.gov/pubmed/24716511

167-http://www.bms.ed.ac.uk/research/others/smaciver/Cyto-Topics/dendritic_spines.htm

168-https://www.ncbi.nlm.nih.gov/pmc/articles/PMC4550756/

169-https://www.ncbi.nlm.nih.gov/pubmed/11706937

170-https://www.ncbi.nlm.nih.gov/pubmed/30703142

171- https://www.amazon.com/Better-Bones-Body-Estrogen-Calcium/dp/0658002899/

172-https://www.ncbi.nlm.nih.gov/pmc/articles/PMC6072880/

173-http://www.ncbi.nlm.nih.gov/pmc/articles/PMC2724665/

174-https://www.ncbi.nlm.nih.gov/pubmed/17350099/

175-https://www.ncbi.nlm.nih.gov/pmc/articles/PMC3471510/

176-https://www.ncbi.nlm.nih.gov/pmc/articles/PMC6072880/

177-https://www.ncbi.nlm.nih.gov/pmc/articles/PMC5938376/

177a- https://www.ncbi.nlm.nih.gov/pmc/articles/PMC3943678/

178-https://www.ncbi.nlm.nih.gov/books/NBK107205/

178a-https://www.ncbi.nlm.nih.gov/pmc/articles/PMC4992603/

179-https://www.ncbi.nlm.nih.gov/pmc/articles/PMC5797832/

179a-https://www.ncbi.nlm.nih.gov/pmc/articles/PMC3943678/

180-https://www.ncbi.nlm.nih.gov/pmc/articles/PMC4634892/

181-https://www.ncbi.nlm.nih.gov/pubmed/27254412

182-https://www.ncbi.nlm.nih.gov/pubmed/22647038

183-https://www.ncbi.nlm.nih.gov/pmc/articles/PMC4604320/

184-https://www.ncbi.nlm.nih.gov/pubmed/24130763

184a- https://www.ncbi.nlm.nih.gov/pmc/articles/PMC5919903/

185-https://www.ncbi.nlm.nih.gov/pmc/articles/PMC3415609/

185a- https://www.sciencedaily.com/releases/
2019/01/190114130825.htm

186-https://www.ncbi.nlm.nih.gov/pmc/articles/PMC4392553/

187-http://www.mdpi.com/1099-4300/15/4/1416

188-www.mdpi.com/1099-4300/15/4/1416

189-https://www.ncbi.nlm.nih.gov/pubmed/29156344

190- https://www.ncbi.nlm.nih.gov/pmc/articles/PMC5550406/

191-https://www.ncbi.nlm.nih.gov/pmc/articles/PMC4538578/

191a-https://www.bmartin.cc/dissent/documents/Samuels13.pdf

192-https://www.ncbi.nlm.nih.gov/pubmed/25801782/

193-https://www.researchgate.net/publication/
261800913_Glyphosate_Its_Effects_on_Humans

194-https://www.ncbi.nlm.nih.gov/pmc/articles/PMC4879184/

195-www.ncbi.nlm.nih.gov/pmc/articles/PMC6630622

196- https://www.ewg.org/news/news-releases/2008/05/13/major-study-
teflon-chemical-people-suggests-harm-immune-system-liver

197-https://www.ncbi.nlm.nih.gov/pmc/articles/PMC5649154/

198-https://www.ncbi.nlm.nih.gov/pmc/articles/PMC3578234/

199-https://www.ncbi.nlm.nih.gov/pmc/articles/PMC5547465/

200-https://www.fda.gov/media/131151/download

201- http://www.nature.com/bdj/journal/v217/n2/full/sj.bdj.2014.606.html

202-https://www.ncbi.nlm.nih.gov/pmc/articles/PMC6427756/

202a- https://www.ncbi.nlm.nih.gov/pubmed/17207072

203-https://www.ncbi.nlm.nih.gov/pmc/articles/PMC4800930/

204-https://www.imt.ie/opinion/letters/link-fluoride-levels-alzheimers-disease-22-02-2018/

205- https://www.healthcentral.com/article/poor-dental-hygiene-linked-to-brain-tissue-degeneration

206-https://www.ncbi.nlm.nih.gov/pmc/articles/PMC3293881/

207-https://www.ncbi.nlm.nih.gov/pmc/articles/PMC3551118/

208-https://www.ncbi.nlm.nih.gov/pubmed/24625052

209-https://www.ncbi.nlm.nih.gov/pubmed/22403632/

210-https://www.ncbi.nlm.nih.gov/pmc/articles/PMC4470692/

211-https://www.ncbi.nlm.nih.gov/pubmed/26200659

212-https://www.ncbi.nlm.nih.gov/pubmed/24440006

213-https://www.ncbi.nlm.nih.gov/pubmed/23657152

214-wwf.panda.org/?22255/Sugar-and-the-Environment-Encouraging-Better-Management-Practices-in-Sugar-Production-and-Processing

215-https://www.ncbi.nlm.nih.gov/pubmed/31095511

216-https://www.ncbi.nlm.nih.gov/pmc/articles/PMC4282293/

217-https://www.ncbi.nlm.nih.gov/pmc/articles/PMC4628075/

218-https://www.ncbi.nlm.nih.gov/pmc/articles/PMC3897598/

219-https://www.ncbi.nlm.nih.gov/pmc/articles/PMC3377298/

220-https://www.ncbi.nlm.nih.gov/pubmed/25345082

221- www.beyondpesticides.org/assets/media/documents/infoservices/
pesticidesandyou/documents/watertesting.pdf

222-https://www.ncbi.nlm.nih.gov/pmc/articles/PMC4144270/

223-www.ncbi.nlm.nih.gov/pubmed/9470898

224-www.jnmjournal.org/journal/view.html?uid=1105&vmd=Full&

225-https://www.ncbi.nlm.nih.gov/pubmed/25779692

225a-https://www.ncbi.nlm.nih.gov/pubmed/15617848

226-journals.plos.org/plospathogens/article?id=10.1371/
journal.ppat.1003726

227-https://www.ncbi.nlm.nih.gov/pubmed/23272543

228-http://www.sciencedaily.com/releases/2016/02/160208083606.htm

229-https://www.ncbi.nlm.nih.gov/books/NBK507256/

230-https://www.ncbi.nlm.nih.gov/books/NBK507256/ see also https://
www.ncbi.nlm.nih.gov/pubmed/20152124

231-https://www.ncbi.nlm.nih.gov/pmc/articles/PMC4425174/

232-https://www.ncbi.nlm.nih.gov/pubmed/22593932

233-https://www.ncbi.nlm.nih.gov/pmc/articles/PMC2763246/

234-https://www.ncbi.nlm.nih.gov/pmc/articles/PMC5562667/

235-https://www.ncbi.nlm.nih.gov/pmc/articles/PMC2249747/

236-https://www.sciencedirect.com/science/article/pii/S0891584913002062

237-https://www.ncbi.nlm.nih.gov/pmc/articles/PMC3640603/

238-https://www.ncbi.nlm.nih.gov/pmc/articles/PMC3057175/

239-https://www.jwatch.org/na31178/2013/06/03/relaxation-response-changes-gene-expression

240-https://www.ncbi.nlm.nih.gov/pmc/articles/PMC4177524/

241a-http://www.cam.ac.uk/research/news/brain-cells-created-from-patients-skin-cells

Psychobiotics
Footnotes:

1-https://www.ncbi.nlm.nih.gov/pmc/articles/PMC4351418/

1a-https://academic.oup.com/jcem/article/89/6/2548/2870285 see also
https://journals.physiology.org/doi/full/10.1152/japplphysiol.00134.2005

2-https://www.ncbi.nlm.nih.gov/pmc/articles/PMC5414803/

3-https://www.livescience.com/63569-gut-bacteria-produces-
electricity.html

4-www.ajmc.com/publications/supplement/2007/2007-11-vol13-
n7Suppl/Nov07-2657pS170-S177/

5-https://www.ncbi.nlm.nih.gov/pubmed/23645137

6-https://www.ncbi.nlm.nih.gov/pmc/articles/PMC6582584/

7-www.cidrap.umn.edu/news-perspective/2018/03/study-non-antibiotic-
drugs-affect-gut-bacteria-could-promote-resistance

8-https://www.ncbi.nlm.nih.gov/pmc/articles/PMC5414803/

9-https://www.ncbi.nlm.nih.gov/pmc/articles/PMC4662178/

10-https://www.amazon.com/Path-Healthy-Mind-Connie-Rogers/dp/
0692566066

11-https://www.sciencedaily.com/releases/2019/06/190623143055.htm

12-https://www.ncbi.nlm.nih.gov/pmc/articles/PMC4315778/

13-www.apa.org/monitor/2012/09/gut-feeling.aspx

14-https://www.ncbi.nlm.nih.gov/pmc/articles/PMC5031164/

15-https://www.ncbi.nlm.nih.gov/pmc/articles/PMC1479485/

16-https://www.ncbi.nlm.nih.gov/pmc/articles/PMC3904694/

17-https://www.ncbi.nlm.nih.gov/pmc/articles/PMC4370913/

18-https://www.drugwatch.com/news/2012/01/22/disease-mongering-and-drug-marketing/

19-allergiesandyourgut.com/tag/psychobiotics/

20-https://ajp.psychiatryonline.org/doi/full/10.1176/appi.ajp.160.3.504

21-https://www.ncbi.nlm.nih.gov/pmc/articles/PMC1275956/

22-https://www.ncbi.nlm.nih.gov/books/NBK519712/table/ch3.t12/

23-https://www.nhs.uk/conditions/social-anxiety/

24-https://en.wikipedia.org/wiki/Emotional_intelligence

25-https://news.rutgers.edu/research-news/label-medication-orders-rise-children/20190911#.XX-O4i2ZMUs

26-https://news.rutgers.edu/research-news/label-medication-orders-rise-children/20190911#.Xg5r9i2ZPyh

27-https://en.wikipedia.org/wiki/National_Institute_of_Mental_Health

28-https://en.wikipedia.org/wiki/Mifepristone

29-https://en.wikipedia.org/wiki/Antidepressant

29a-https://www.rxlist.com/script/main/art.asp?articlekey=17889

30-https://en.wikipedia.org/wiki/Mental_illness

31-https://dailybruin.com/2013/03/01/ucla-researchers-discover-new-drug-that-alleviates-anxiety/

32-https://www.drugs.com/mtm/scopolamine.html

33-https://www.drugs.com/paroxetine.html

34-https://clinicaltrials.gov/ct2/show/NCT03664232

35-https://en.wikipedia.org/wiki/JNJ-42165279

36-https://www.fiercebiotech.com/r-d/j-j-halts-a-depression-program-shadow-of-a-fatal-french-trial

37-https://www.nimh.nih.gov/health/publications/social-anxiety-disorder-more-than-just-shyness/19-mh-8083-socialanxietydisordermorethanjustshyness_153750.pdf

38-www.nimh.nih.gov/health/topics/anxiety-disorders/index.shtml

39-https://www.madinamerica.com/author/kbrogan/

40-www.greenmedinfo.com/blog/depression-it-s-not-your-serotonin

41-https://www.ncbi.nlm.nih.gov/pubmed/17207972

42-https://www.ncbi.nlm.nih.gov/pubmed/23759244

43-https://www.ncbi.nlm.nih.gov/pubmed/27621125

44-https://www.ncbi.nlm.nih.gov/pmc/articles/PMC4822287/

45-https://www.ncbi.nlm.nih.gov/pubmed/23441623

46-https://www.ncbi.nlm.nih.gov/pubmed/30056107

47-https://www.ncbi.nlm.nih.gov/pubmed/30125859

48-https://www.ncbi.nlm.nih.gov/books/NBK92775/

49-https://www.ncbi.nlm.nih.gov/pmc/articles/PMC5102282/

50-https://medicalxpress.com/news/2016-10-current-state-psychobiotics.html

51-https://www.ncbi.nlm.nih.gov/pmc/articles/PMC4471960/

52-https://www.ncbi.nlm.nih.gov/pmc/articles/PMC4980946/

53-https://www.cell.com/trends/neurosciences/fulltext/S0166-2236(16)30113-8

53a- https://www.ncbi.nlm.nih.gov/pmc/articles/PMC1479485/

54-https://www.sciencedirect.com/science/article/pii/S2352289516300509

55-https://www.ncbi.nlm.nih.gov/pmc/articles/PMC4500982/

56-https://en.wikipedia.org/wiki/Lactobacillus_rhamnosus

57-https://www.drugs.com/mtm/lactobacillus-rhamnosus-gg.html

58-https://bpspubs.onlinelibrary.wiley.com/doi/10.1111/bph.14127

59-https://new.hindawi.com/journals/tswj/2014/780616/

60-https://www.ncbi.nlm.nih.gov/pmc/articles/PMC181180/

61-https://www.ncbi.nlm.nih.gov/pmc/articles/PMC2723593/

62-https://www.ncbi.nlm.nih.gov/pubmed/29777524

63-www.scielo.br/scielo.php?script=sci_arttext&pid=S0100-879X1997001200003

64-onlinelibrary.wiley.com/doi/10.1111/j.1749-6632.2012.06569.x/full

65-https://www.ncbi.nlm.nih.gov/pmc/articles/PMC2858344/

66-https://www.ncbi.nlm.nih.gov/pubmed/23847492

67-www.brainfacts.org/across-the-lifespan/stress-and-anxiety/articles/2012/stress-the-role-of-glucocorticoids/

68-https://www.ncbi.nlm.nih.gov/pmc/articles/PMC4662771/

69-https://www.ncbi.nlm.nih.gov/pubmed/21322550

70- www.scielo.br/scielo.php?pid=S0101-81082005000200008&script=sci_arttext&tlng=en

71-www.mdedge.com/currentpsychiatry/article/62206/corticosteroid-induced-mania-prepare-unpredictable

72-https://www.mayoclinicproceedings.org/article/S0025-6196(11)61160-9/pdf

73-https://www.sciencedirect.com/science/article/pii/S0361923018303678

74-https://www.ncbi.nlm.nih.gov/books/NBK531462/

75-https://www.ncbi.nlm.nih.gov/pmc/articles/PMC3934796/

76-https://www.ncbi.nlm.nih.gov/pmc/articles/PMC4857870/

77-https://www.ncbi.nlm.nih.gov/pmc/articles/PMC4207041/

78-https://ajp.psychiatryonline.org/doi/full/10.1176/appi.ajp.2014.14010008

79-https://www.ncbi.nlm.nih.gov/pmc/articles/PMC4315778/

80-https://www.nature.com/scitable/topicpage/epigenetic-influences-and-disease-895/

81-https://www.ncbi.nlm.nih.gov/pubmed/28691768

82-https://www.ncbi.nlm.nih.gov/pubmed/23150270

83-https://jme.bioscientifica.com/view/journals/jme/60/2/JME-17-0189.xml

84-https://www.nature.com/articles/mp2016192

85-https://www.ncbi.nlm.nih.gov/pmc/articles/PMC4762453/

86-https://www.ncbi.nlm.nih.gov/pubmed/30718923

87-www.sigmaaldrich.com/catalog/product/sigma/d1756?lang=en&region=US

88-www.everydayhealth.com/drugs/prozac

89-www.iodine.com/drug/prozac

90-https://www.lilly.com/who-we-are/governance/board-of-directors

91-https://www.bloomberg.com/news/articles/2017-06-12/basf-syngenta-said-among-bidders-for-bayer-monsanto-disposals

92-injury.findlaw.com/product-liability/atrazine-lawsuit-overview.html

93-https://journals.plos.org/plosone/article?id=10.1371/journal.pone.0184306

94-www.ncbi.nlm.nih.gov/pmc/articles/PMC4228144/

95-https://spinalresearch.com.au/kills-gut-bacteria-kill-brain-cells-new-study-critiques-prolonged-antibiotic-use/

96-https://www.sciencedaily.com/releases/2016/05/160519130105.htm

97-https://www.frontiersin.org/articles/10.3389/fpsyt.2018.00776/full#B21

98-https://www.ncbi.nlm.nih.gov/pubmed/20352091

99-www.actionbioscience.org/evolution/meade_callahan.html

100-www.madehow.com/knowledge/Ammonia.html

101-www.thefreedictionary.com/Saprophytic+bacteria

102-https://www.ncbi.nlm.nih.gov/pmc/articles/PMC3927245/

103-https://www.ncbi.nlm.nih.gov/pubmed/18425703

104-https://jamanetwork.com/journals/jamaneurology/fullarticle/777652

105-https://academic.oup.com/alcalc/article/47/5/497/98894/Alterations-of-Homocysteine-Serum-Levels-during

105a-https://www.ncbi.nlm.nih.gov/pmc/articles/PMC4069007/

106-https://www.medpagetoday.com/primarycare/obesity/82412

106a- https://www.ncbi.nlm.nih.gov/pmc/articles/PMC2685204/

107-www.alternet.org/food/monsantos-roundup-weedkiller-changes-dna-function-causing-chronic-disease

108-https://ehjournal.biomedcentral.com/articles/10.1186/s12940-018-0367-0

109-journals.plos.org/plospathogens/article?id=10.1371/journal.ppat.1003726

110-https://www.ncbi.nlm.nih.gov/pmc/articles/PMC3697199/

111-https://www.ncbi.nlm.nih.gov/pubmed/11972140

112-https://www.ncbi.nlm.nih.gov/pmc/articles/PMC3218792/

113-https://www.ncbi.nlm.nih.gov/pmc/articles/PMC3632337/

114-https://en.wikipedia.org/wiki/Corcept_Therapeutics

114a-https://www.rxlist.com/contrave-side-effects-drug-center.htm#overview

115-https://ajp.psychiatryonline.org/doi/full/10.1176/appi.ajp.2014.14010008

116-https://www.ncbi.nlm.nih.gov/pmc/articles/PMC3181883/

117-https://www.ncbi.nlm.nih.gov/pubmed/2769898/

118-europepmc.org/articles/pmc4673005

119-www.ncbi.nlm.nih.gov/pubmed/15929893

120-www.ncbi.nlm.nih.gov/pubmed/17218051

121-https://www.bmj.com/content/363/bmj.k4576/rr-1

122-https://www.naturalnewsblogs.com/sick-toxic/

123-https://www.ncbi.nlm.nih.gov/books/NBK19961/

124-https://www.ncbi.nlm.nih.gov/pubmed/24088149

125-www.realfarmacy.com/mental-nutrition/

Prevent Kidney Disorders -
Footnotes:

1- https://www.mdanderson.org/newsroom/potential-new-therapy-approaches-to-reverse-kidney-damage-identi.h00-158989812.html

2- https://www.ncbi.nlm.nih.gov/pubmed/26149669/

3- https://www.ncbi.nlm.nih.gov/pmc/articles/PMC4641625/

4- www.encyclopedia.com/medicine/diseases-and-conditions/pathology/insulin-resistance

5- https://www.ncbi.nlm.nih.gov/pmc/articles/PMC6071166/

6- https://www.ncbi.nlm.nih.gov/pmc/articles/PMC3820526/

7- https://jamanetwork.com/journals/jama/fullarticle/199317

8- https://www.ncbi.nlm.nih.gov/pmc/articles/PMC3299001/

9- https://www.ncbi.nlm.nih.gov/pmc/articles/PMC4263906/

10- https://www.ncbi.nlm.nih.gov/pubmed/9415946/

11- https://www.drlamcoaching.com/blog/insomnia-and-adrenal-fatigue/

12- https://www.drlam.com/articles/adrenal_fatigue.asp

13- https://www.sciencedaily.com/releases/2016/11/161129143428.htm

14- https://www.ncbi.nlm.nih.gov/pmc/articles/PMC4323914/

15- https://www.ncbi.nlm.nih.gov/pmc/articles/PMC4561915/

16- https://www.ncbi.nlm.nih.gov/pmc/articles/PMC6024687/

17- https://www.healthline.com/health/sertraline-oral-tablet

18- https://www.economist.com/business/2019/05/30/johnson-and-johnson-stands-trial-for-the-opioid-crisis?

19- https://www.rxlist.com/humira-side-effects-drug-center.htm#overview

20- https://www.ehealthme.com/ds/abilify/chronic-kidney-disease/

21- https://www.avastin.com/patient/mcrc/treatment/possible-side-effects.html

21a-https://www.drugwatch.com/news/2017/05/11/fda-cancer-warning-antacids/

21b=https://www.drugwatch.com/proton-pump-inhibitors/prilosec/

22- https://academic.oup.com/ndt/article/24/12/3582/1833083

23- https://www.acufinder.com/Acupuncture+Information/Detail/Healthy+Eyes+with+Chinese+Medicine

24- https://www.ncbi.nlm.nih.gov/pmc/articles/PMC3247860/

25- https://www.sciencedaily.com/releases/2009/10/091010120051.htm

26- www.healnatl.org/gulf-war-veterans-illnesses-toxic-exposures-pesticides-used-gulf/

27- visitwww.vaclib.org/basic/contamination/medcrave.htm

28- https://www.ncbi.nlm.nih.gov/pmc/articles/PMC5454951/

29- https://www.ncbi.nlm.nih.gov/pmc/articles/PMC4934868/

30- https://www.intechopen.com/books/chronic-kidney-disease-from-pathophysiology-to-clinical-improvements/role-of-organochlorine-pesticides-in-chronic-kidney-diseases-of-unknown-etiology

31- https://bmjopen.bmj.com/content/6/7/e011836

32- https://cjasn.asnjournals.org/content/6/1/218

33- https://onlinelibrary.wiley.com/doi/abs/10.1111/nep.13225?af=R

34- https://www.health.ny.gov/prevention/dental/impact_oral_health.htm

35- https://www.ncbi.nlm.nih.gov/pmc/articles/PMC6221676/

36- https://journals.lww.com/md-journal/Fulltext/2018/11020/
The_association_between_BMI_and_kidney_cancer.16.aspx#R17-16

37- https://www.ncbi.nlm.nih.gov/pmc/articles/PMC3407016/

38- https://www.ncbi.nlm.nih.gov/pmc/articles/PMC4194023/

39- https://www.ncbi.nlm.nih.gov/pubmed/25763405

40- https://www.ncbi.nlm.nih.gov/pmc/articles/PMC5920374/

41- www.emfwise.com/science_details.php

42- https://www.ncbi.nlm.nih.gov/pmc/articles/PMC5014506/

43- https://link.springer.com/article/10.1007/s00467-016-3392-7

44- https://www.ncbi.nlm.nih.gov/pmc/articles/PMC4491063/

45- https://www.ncbi.nlm.nih.gov/pmc/articles/PMC3169868/

46- https://www.ncbi.nlm.nih.gov/pmc/articles/PMC3313737/

46a-https://www.ncbi.nlm.nih.gov/pubmed/23239393

46b-https://www.ncbi.nlm.nih.gov/pmc/articles/PMC4070857/

46c-https://www.ncbi.nlm.nih.gov/pmc/articles/PMC6146775/

47- https://www.medicalnewstoday.com/articles/318415.php

48- https://www.omicsonline.org/open-access/glyphosate-substitution-for-glycine-during-protein-synthesis-as-a-causal-factor-in-mesoamerican-nephropathy-2161-0525-1000541-99002.html

49- https://sustainablepulse.com/2014/11/07/new-study-huge-increase-us-chronic-diseases-linked-glyphosate-herbicides/#.XSvRRGVR5zi

50- www.scirp.org/reference/ReferencesPapers.aspx? ReferenceID=1639107

51- jphe.amegroups.com/article/view/3665/4415

52- https://www.ncbi.nlm.nih.gov/pubmed/25635985?dopt=Abstract

53-https://www.thelancet.com/commissions/pollution-and-health

53a- https://beyondpesticides.org/dailynewsblog/2016/07/glyphosate-causes-changes-dna-resulting-chronic-disease/

54- https://neurosciencenews.com/lymphatic-system-brain-neurobiology-2080/

53- https://www.ackdjournal.org/article/S1548-5595(10)00054-6/fulltext

54-https://www.ncbi.nlm.nih.gov/pmc/articles/PMC4957724/

55- https://www.ncbi.nlm.nih.gov/pmc/articles/PMC5907783/

To contact the author please visit BiteSizePieces.net

Printed in the United States of America.

ISBN: 978-0-578-65119-4

Made in the USA
Columbia, SC
07 March 2020